Psoriasis - New Research

Edited by Shahin Aghaei

Published in London, United Kingdom

Psoriasis - New Research
http://dx.doi.org/10.5772/intechopen.96838
Edited by Shahin Aghaei

Contributors
Aylin Turel Ermertcan, Ece Gokyayla, Tubanur Cetinarslan, Ian P. Harrison, Dalibor Mijaljica, Fabrizio Spada, Suxing Liu, Weikang Tao, Di Li, Seema Chhabra, Lekha Rani, Smrity Sahu, Keshav Sharma, Maryada Sharma, Ranjana Minz, Sunil Dogra, Naoki Kondo, Rika Kakutani, Masahiko Yamada, Tamilselvi Elango, Anburaj Jeyaraj, Haripriya Dayalan, Xinghui Li, Pushpa Gnanaraj, Xuejun Zhang, Florentina Silvia Delli, Elena Sotiriou, Monica Neagu, Mihaela Surcel, Carolina Constantin, Adriana Narcisa Munteanu

First published in London, United Kingdom, 2022 by IntechOpen
IntechOpen is the global imprint of INTECHOPEN LIMITED, registered in England and Wales, registration number: 11086078, 5 Princes Gate Court, London, SW7 2QJ, United Kingdom

British Library Cataloguing-in-Publication Data
A catalogue record for this book is available from the British Library

Additional hard and PDF copies can be obtained from orders@intechopen.com

Psoriasis - New Research
Edited by Shahin Aghaei
p. cm.
Print ISBN 978-1-80355-375-7
Online ISBN 978-1-80355-376-4
eBook (PDF) ISBN 978-1-80355-377-1

Meet the editor

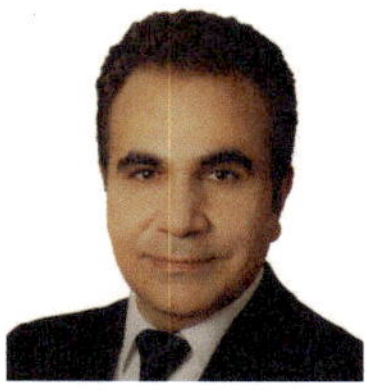

Shahin Aghaei, MD, graduated from Shiraz University of Medical Sciences, Iran, in 2004. He was awarded a fellowship from the International Society of Dermatopathology (ISD) from Charles University, Czech Republic, in 2008 and a fellowship in Dermatologic Surgery from the Medical University of Graz, Austria, in 2010. He is currently editor in chief of the *Journal of Surgical Dermatology* in Singapore and Associate Professor of Dermatology and Dermatologic Surgery at Iran University of Medical Sciences, School of Medicine. He is also a member of the American Academy of Dermatology, European Academy of Dermatology and Venereology, American Society for Laser Medicine and Surgery, International Society of Dermatology, International Hyperhidrosis Society, and Iranian Society of Dermatology.

Contents

Preface

Psoriasis is an autoimmune disease that causes rapid accumulation of skin cells. This accumulation causes well-demarcated, raised, silver-white, scaly lesions to appear on the surface of the skin such as the scalp, elbows and knees, genitalia, and nails. The prevalence of psoriasis in the United States is about 2% of the total population. This disease is always related to other diseases and the affected person may also have one of the following: type 2 diabetes, inflammatory bowel disease, heart disease, psoriatic arthritis, anxiety, or depression. This book reviews recent literature on the most significant and important studies about psoriasis, the immunological mechanisms involved, the latest dermoscopic and diagnostic methods, and recent methods of treatments. This book includes three sections and eight chapters.

Section 1: "Clinical Criteria, Differential Diagnosis and Comorbidities"

Chapter 1: "The Clinical Characteristics and Treatment Status of Psoriatic Arthritis"

Psoriatic arthritis (PsA) is a complex musculoskeletal disorder. Its clinical features include psoriasis, peripheral arthritis, spinal involvement, enthesitis, and dactylitis. Typically, skin lesions precede osteoarticular lesions, although osteoarticular lesions can precede skin lesions in some cases. This chapter investigates the onset pattern of PsA, the time interval between the occurrence of skin and osteoarticular lesions, and the treatment status of PsA. The study presented in this chapter included sixty-four patients with PsA who had been assessed according to the CASPAR criteria. Of those patients, 75% had a typical lesion-onset pattern where skin lesions preceded osteoarticular lesions (skin leading) and 16% had an osteoarticular-leading lesion pattern. The mean time interval between the onset of lesions in patients with the skin-leading pattern was 14.2 years and that in patients with the osteoarticular-leading pattern was 4.5 years. Non-steroidal anti-inflammatory drugs were prescribed to 39% of patients, conventional synthetic disease-modifying antirheumatic drugs (DMARDs) to 64%, and biologic DMARDs to 51.5%. Because there were several cases where osteoarticular lesions preceded skin lesions in PsA, the chapter authors suggest care should be taken with regard to oligo- or polyarthritis patients with a negative rheumatoid factor without the presence of skin lesions.

Chapter 2: "Dermoscopic Differential Diagnosis of Psoriasis"

Different clinical subtypes of psoriasis can show distinctive clinical appearances. For example, inverse psoriasis does not have squams and resembles erythema intertrigo and sometimes the erythrodermic variant cannot be distinguished from other erythroderma causes. As such, differential diagnosis of psoriasis should be done carefully to manage the disease appropriately. Histopathological examination is the gold standard technique for diagnosis, but a dermatoscope can also be used. This is a non-invasive and easily applicable diagnostic tool with high specificity. This chapter discusses the dermoscopic differential diagnosis of psoriasis.

Chapter 3: "Psoriasis and Skin Comorbidities"

Psoriasis can have many clinical presentations in patients with different medical backgrounds. Medical specialties such as rheumatology, pathology, and cardiology focus on the systemic inflammatory nature of the psoriatic disease. From a dermatological point of view, skin comorbidities are an important issue that affects therapeutic choice. The common comorbidities with psoriasis include vitiligo, alopecia areata, autoimmune bullous skin diseases like bullous pemphigoid and pemphigus vulgaris, and other skin disorders such as hidradenitis suppurativa, and pityriasis rubra pilaris. One of the most paradoxical relationships is between psoriasis and atopic dermatitis. This chapter discusses and describes various comorbidities of psoriasis.

Section 2: "Immune System and Psoriasis"

Chapter 4: "Th17/IL-17, Immunometabolism and Psoriatic Disease: A Pathological Trifecta"

The burgeoning arena of immunometabolism provides evidence of the role of cellular as well as local (tissue)/systemic metabolic pathways in controlling immunity and inflammation. An intricate and elaborate network of various metabolic circuits, specifically glycolysis, fatty acid oxidation and synthesis, and amino acid metabolism, precisely generates metabolites that rewire the immune response. Psoriasis is a chronic progressive self-perpetuated "IL-17-centric" inflammatory disease characterized by the co-existence of autoimmune and autoinflammatory pathways. Metabolic responses, governed by oxygen levels, nutrient availability, growth factors, cytokines, AMP/ATP ratios, and amino acids, play a pivotal role in programming Th17 cell fate determination. Understanding the intricate interactions and complex interplay of molecular mechanisms responsible for Th17 cell metabolic rewiring, an important determinant of Th17 cell plasticity and heterogeneity, has the potential to reshape psoriatic therapeutics in ways currently unimagined. This chapter presents recent updates on major cellular and systemic metabolic pathways regulating differentiation of Th17 cells as well their crosstalk with intracellular signaling mediators. It also sheds light on how dysregulation of these pathways can be responsible for immune impairment and the development of psoriatic disease. A better understanding of these metabolic processes could unveil an intriguing leverage point for therapeutic interventions to modulate metabolic programming and Th17 cell responses in this multisystemic inflammatory disease.

Chapter 5: "Immune Markers in Psoriasis"

Psoriasis is a chronic inflammatory skin disorder with high immunological background caused by a complex interplay between an altered immune system, genetic factors, autoantigens, lifestyle, and environmental factors. Extensive literature in recent years has highlighted the crucial role played by the immune system in the pathogenesis of this pathology. Although it is unequivocally accepted that psoriasis is a T-cell-mediated autoimmune condition, both innate and specific immune cells are highly involved in its pathogenesis. The aberrant interactions between immune cells and resident hyper-proliferative keratinocytes are mediated by immune- and non-immune-related molecules that lead to amplification of the local immune responses that maintain the chronic inflammatory status. This chapter discusses the immune molecules residing in the psoriatic tissue or appending to the blood circulation that can indicate the prognosis of this systemic autoimmune disease. It also focuses on residing or circulating immune cells that can pinpoint the clinical evolution of the psoriatic disease. All these data can be developed in immune marker patterns that aid psoriasis diagnosis and/or future (immune)therapies.

Chapter 6 "Immunomodulatory Effect of Methotrexate Abruptly Controls Keratinocyte Activation in Psoriasis"

In psoriatic skin, epidermal keratinocytes undergo deregulated inflammatory response that leads to prolonged expression of inflammatory mediators as well as abnormal keratins. Due to immune and genetic factors, keratinocytes get activated and cell balance gets disturbed. This activation is mainly due to deregulated inflammatory response. A vicious cycle of keratinocyte-immune response called the keratinocyte activation cycle leads to psoriasis in psoriatic skin. Epidermal keratinocytes undergo deregulated inflammatory response that leads to prolonged expression of inflammatory mediators as well as abnormal keratins. Methotrexate, an immunosuppressive agent, has been used as a standard drug to treat severe psoriasis. Acanthosis and abnormal terminal differentiation were mainly due to the mutation in epidermal keratins. In turn, disease severity and relapsing of psoriasis are mainly due to the mutation of hyperproliferative keratins. These novel keratin mutations in psoriatic epidermis might be one of the causative factors for psoriasis. Methotrexate strongly regulates the keratinocyte activation cycle by deregulated inflammatory markers and maintains a normal keratin phenotype on hyperproliferating keratinocytes, thereby controlling acanthosis in psoriasis patients.

Section 3: "Treatment of Psoriasis"

Chapter 7: "Topical Moisturisers for the Management of Psoriasis Vulgaris"

This chapter provides an overview of basic and tailored topical moisturizers and discusses how and why they form the backbone for the management of psoriasis. The discussion begins by describing the main characteristics of psoriasis and indicating how alterations in the skin's integrity and barrier function contribute to the initial development of psoriasis and subsequent changes in psoriasis phenotype. Next, the chapter addresses the evolution of topical moisturizers to more sophisticated and beneficial products and describes the key biophysical effects exerted on psoriatic skin by their active ingredients as well as the myriad benefits offered by fundamental and specialty ingredients. Furthermore, the chapter explains how topical moisturizer formulation modalities can help to improve compromised skin barrier function and alleviate the symptoms of psoriasis, cosmetically and/or therapeutically. It also discusses associated concerns and challenges.

Chapter 8 "Developing Novel Molecular Targeted Therapeutics for Topical Treatment of Psoriasis"

In mild-to-moderate as well as moderate-to-severe psoriasis, 70%–80% of patients start with topical agents and continue to use them with other active therapies. This group of patients can benefit from topical treatment with minimal systemic exposure. The expression levels of IL-23 and IL-17 are upregulated in psoriatic skin compared with non-lesional skin. Epidermal proliferation and psoriasis are caused by overactive Th17 cells, which are promoted and stabilized by the activated IL-23 receptor, forming part of the positive feedback loop. FDA-approved biologics in IL-23/IL-17 axis (ustekinumab, guselkumab, risankizumab, tildrakizumab, ixekizumab, secukinumab, and brodalumab) demonstrated superior clinical efficacy in the systemic treatment of moderate-to-severe psoriasis, providing clinical proof of the IL-23/IL-17 axis as a major immune pathway underlying the pathophysiology of psoriasis. However, due to its large size and poor permeability to the skin, biologics are not suitable to deliver via topical route. Current topical treatments of mild-to-moderate psoriasis are corticosteroids and vitamin D analogues, which have limited efficacy with significant side effects so patients must avoid long-term use. This chapter reviews current molecular targeted therapeutics under development for topical treatment of psoriasis.

Shahin Aghaei, MD
Department of Dermatology and Dermatological Surgery,
Iran University of Medical Sciences,
Tehran, Iran

Section 1

Clinical Criteria, Differential Diagnosis and Comorbidities

Chapter 1

The Clinical Characteristics and Treatment Status of Psoriatic Arthritis

Naoki Kondo, Masahiko Yamada and Rika Kakutani

Abstract

Psoriatic arthritis (PsA) is a complex musculoskeletal disorder. Its clinical features include psoriasis, peripheral arthritis, spinal involvement, enthesitis, and dactylitis. Typically, skin lesions precede osteoarticular lesions, although osteoarticular lesions can precede skin lesions in some cases. This study aimed to investigate the onset pattern of PsA, the time interval between the occurrence of skin and osteoarticular lesions, and the treatment status of PsA. A total of 64 patients with PsA who had been assessed according to the CASPAR criteria were enrolled. Of those, 75% had a typical lesion onset pattern where skin lesions preceded osteoarticular lesions (skin leading) and 16% had an osteoarticular leading lesion pattern. The mean time interval between the onset of lesions in patients with the skin leading pattern was 14.2 years and that in patients with the osteoarticular leading pattern was 4.5 years. Non-steroidal anti-inflammatory drugs were prescribed to 39% of patients, conventional synthetic disease modifying antirheumatic drugs (DMARDs) to 64%, and biologic DMARDs to 51.5%. In conclusion, there were several cases where osteoarticular lesions preceded skin lesions in PsA; therefore, care should be taken with regard to oligo- or poly-arthritis patients with a negative rheumatoid factor without the presence of skin lesions.

Keywords: bDMARDs, CASPAR criteria, csDMARDs, obesity, psoriatic arthritis

1. Introduction

Psoriatic arthritis (PsA) is a complex musculoskeletal disorder that has the clinical features of psoriasis, peripheral arthritis, spinal involvement, enthesitis, and dactylitis [1, 2]. Typically, skin lesions precede osteoarticular lesions [1–6], although osteoarticular lesions precede skin lesions in some cases. In these cases, the diagnosis is difficult and often results in a delay in treatment. Regardless, the appropriate management of PsA requires early diagnosis. Classification criteria of PsA (CASPAR criteria) consist of established inflammatory articular diseases with at least 3 points from the following features: current psoriasis (assigned a score of 2), a history of psoriasis (a score of 1), a family history of psoriasis (a score of 1), dactylitis (a score of 1), juxtaarticular new bone formation (a score of 1), rheumatoid factor negativity (a score of 1), and nail dystrophy (a score of 1). The CASPAR criteria have been reported to be useful in assisting clinicians in the diagnosis of PsA because of high sensitivity and specificity than any other criteria [7].

PsA in many patients is associated with obesity, diabetes, hypertension, metabolic syndrome, fatty liver, and an increased risk of cardiovascular events compared to that of the general population [8]. In a realistic orthopedic outpatient clinical setting, little is unknown about the clinical features and the treatment status in patients with PsA. Whether PsA is associated with obesity or lifestyle-related diseases remains unknown.

We investigated the clinical characteristics of PsA, such as the onset pattern of PsA, the interval between the occurrence of skin lesions and osteoarticular lesions, and the distribution of arthritis such as peripheral and axial lesions and enthesitis. In addition, we examined whether obesity, hypertension, or diabetes mellitus was significantly increased in patients with PsA. We also examined the treatment status for PsA.

2. Methods

This was a single-center non-interventional retrospective study that examined patients with PsA who were diagnosed by rheumatologists and dermatologists at our hospital between January 2010 and December 2018. All patients in this study satisfied the CASPAR criteria with a score of more than 3 points. A total of 64 consecutive cases were enrolled, and informed consent was obtained from each patient. This study was approved by Niigata University Medical and Dental Hospital Institutional Review Board (#2018–0418).

The patients were categorized and investigated according to the following PsA onset patterns: a skin rash that preceded the manifestations of arthritis (skin leading type), the osteoarticular lesion that preceded the manifestation of a skin rash (osteoarticular leading type), and the simultaneous onset of skin and osteoarticular symptoms (simultaneous type). For both the skin and osteoarticular leading types of PsA, we recorded the time between the presentation of the first and second symptoms. We also investigated the disease prevalence according to the lesion site, namely peripheral lesions (e.g., fingers, wrists, elbows, shoulders, toes, ankles, knees, and hips), axial lesions (e.g., cervical, thoracic, lumbar spines, and sacroiliac joint), and enthesitis (e.g., Achilles' tendon, plantar aponeurosis, quadriceps tendon, and patellar tendon).

When arthritis symptoms were present, painful areas were evaluated by radiography, which allowed us to confirm the presence of imaging findings typical of PsA (typical peripheral joint new bone formation, sacroiliac joint bone erosions, and syndesmophytes on the sacroiliac joint or spine).

Obesity was defined as a body mass index (BMI) ≥ 25, and the prevalence of comorbidities was assessed relative to that of the general population as reported in a survey conducted by the Ministry of Health, Labor, and Welfare of Japan [9]. The incidences of obesity and hypertension, diabetes mellitus, and other diseases such as dyslipidemia and chronic kidney disease were examined.

Furthermore, we classified the patients according to the treatments they had received, such as nonsteroidal anti-inflammatory drugs (NSAIDs), conventional synthetic disease-modifying antirheumatic drugs (csDMARDs), biological DMARDs (bDMARDs), prednisolone, and others.

2.1 Statistical analysis

The statistical analyses were performed using SPSS (Version 21, Tokyo, Japan). The Student t-test was performed for continuous variables, and Fisher's exact probability test was performed for categorical variables. A p-value <0.05 was considered to be statistically significant.

3. Results

Of the 64 patients with PsA who were enrolled, 49 were male and 15 were female patients. The patient characteristics are shown in **Table 1**. The mean age ± SD of the patients was 55.5 ± 12.9 years (range, 27–80 years), and the mean age at the onset of first symptoms was 36.2 ± 15.7 years (range, 3–70 years). The mean age of the onset of psoriasis (skin lesion) and the osteoarticular lesion was 36.2 years and 47.0 years, respectively. The mean time interval between the onset of skin and osteoarticular lesions was 11.3 years (range, 0–39 years). Regarding the CASPAR criteria, the percentage of confirmed items was 100% for current psoriasis, followed by rheumatoid factor negativity (92.4%), nail lesions (34.8%), juxta-articular new bone formation (25.8%), and dactylitis (16.7%); the mean CASPAR score was 3.75 points (range, 3–6 points).

Regarding the onset patterns of PsA, the skin leading type was dominant in 48 cases (75%), with 10 cases of the osteoarticular leading type (15.6%), followed by 6 cases of the simultaneous type (9.4%). The mean time interval between the presentation of the two different lesion types was 14.2 ± 10.2 years (range, 0.3–39.4 years) in the skin leading type and 4.5 ± 3.3 (range, 0.1–15.1 years) in the osteoarticular leading type. A statistically significant difference ($p < 0.001$) was observed between the

Demographic and clinical characteristics (n = 64)	Value (range, %)
Demographic characteristics	
Sex, male/female	49/15
Age	55.5 ± 12.9 years (27–80)
Age at onset of symptoms	36.2 ± 15.7 years (3–70)
Age at psoriasis onset	36.8 years (3–70)
Age at arthritis onset	47.0 years (17–75)
The mean interval between the occurrence of skin lesion and arthritis	11.3 years (0–39)
CASPAR criteria	
Current psoriasis	64 (100)
Dactylitis	11 (16.7)
Juxta-articular new bone formation	17 (25.8)
Rheumatoid factor negativity	61 (92.4)
Typical psoriatic nail lesions	23 (34.8)
Average score	3.75 (3–6)

Table 1.
Characteristics of patients with psoriatic arthritis.

two types (**Table 2**). In addition, no statistically significant difference was observed between the patient's sex and age.

Axial joints were affected in 29% of those in the skin leading group and 60% of the patients in the osteoarticular leading group, although there was no statistically significant difference in the distribution patterns of the affected axial joints ($p = 0.16$). Axial lesions were observed in a total of 21 cases (53%), with the sacroiliac joints the most affected joints in 14 cases (22%), followed by the thoracic spine in 10 cases (16%), lumbar spine in 9 cases (14%), and cervical spine in 7 cases (11%) (**Table 3**).

Peripheral joints were affected in 92% of the patients in the skin leading type and 100% of the patients in the osteoarticular leading type, without a statistically significant difference ($p = 0.99$). Regarding the peripheral joint lesions, 53 cases (83%) were observed in the upper extremity and 30 cases (47%) in the lower extremity. In the upper extremity, the joints that were first affected joint were the finger joints in 39 cases (61%), followed by shoulder joints in 22 cases (34%), wrist joints in 12 cases (19%), and elbow joints in 7 cases (11%). In the lower extremity, the joints that were first affected were the toe joints in 12 cases (19%), followed by knee joints in 11 cases (17%), hip joints in 7 cases (11%), and ankle joints in 4 cases (6.3%) (**Table 4**).

Enthesitis was observed in 15 of the total cases (23%). The most affected tendons were the Achilles' and plantar tendons, both with 8 cases (13%), followed by the quadriceps tendon in 6 cases (9.4%) and patellar tendon in 2 cases (3.1%) (**Table 5**).

In our study, the prevalence of obesity was determined to be 55%. Regarding other comorbid lifestyle-related diseases, hypertension was observed in 27 cases (42%), diabetes mellitus in 12 cases (19%), dyslipidemia in 11 cases (17%), and chronic

Timing of onset	**n or years (range, %)**
Skin leading type	48 (75)
Time interval between the occurrence of skin and osteoarticular lesions	14.2 ± 10.2 years (0.3–39.4)
Simultaneous type	6 (9.4)
Osteoarticular leading type	10 (15.6)
Time interval between the occurrence of osteoarticular and skin lesions	4.5 ± 3.3 (0.1–15.1)*

**shows statistically significant difference ($p < 0.0001$) compared to that of the time interval between the occurrence of skin and osteoarticular lesions.*

Table 2.
The onset patterns of psoriatic arthritis.

The site of axial lesions	**Cases**	**%**
Cervical spine	7	11
Thoracic spine	10	16
Lumbar spine	9	14
Sacroiliac joints	14	22
Total	21	33

Table 3.
The distribution pattern of axial lesions.

Site of peripheral lesions	Cases	%
Upper extremity	53	83
Finger	39	61
Wrist	12	19
Elbow	7	11
Shoulder	22	34
Lower extremity	30	47
Toe	12	19
Ankle	4	6.3
Knee	11	17
Hip	7	11

Table 4.
The distribution pattern of the peripheral lesions.

Site of enthesitis	Cases	%
Achilles' tendon	8	13
Plantar tendon	8	13
Quadriceps tendon	6	9.4
Patellar tendon	2	3.1
Total	15	23

Table 5.
The distribution pattern of enthesitis.

	Present study (%)	Japanese cohort in 2016 (%)	p-value
Obesity (BMI ≥ 25)	55	26	< 0.001
Hypertension	42	36	0.43
Diabetes mellitus	19	15	0.57

Fisher's direct exact test was performed for each patient for obesity and concomitant diseases.
BMI, body mass index.

Table 6.
The incidence of obesity, hypertension, and diabetes mellitus in patients with psoriatic arthritis and comparison with a Japanese cohort.

kidney disease (CKD) in 3 cases (4.7%). Diabetes mellitus was type 2 in all 12 cases. A statistically significant correlation was found between PsA and obesity ($p < 0.0001$). No statistically significant correlations were observed between PsA and hypertension ($p = 0.43$) or diabetes mellitus ($p = 0.57$) (**Table 6**).

Table 7 shows the treatments the patients with PsA received. NSAIDs were prescribed in 25 cases (39%). Several csDMARDs were prescribed in 41 cases (64%), where 21 cases (32.8%) received methotrexate, 9 cases (14%) received salazosulfapyridine, and 3 cases (4.7%) received cyclosporine. Several bDMARDs were prescribed in 33 cases (51.5%), with the most prescribed bDMARDs being

Drug	Cases	%
NSAIDs	25	**39.0**
csDMARDs	**41**	**64.0**
Methotrexate	21	32.8
Salazosulfapyridine	9	14.0
Cyclosporine	3	4.7
Others	6	9.4
bDMARDs	**33**	**51.5**
Adalimumab	10	15.6
Infliximab	10	15.6
Etanercept	3	4.7
Certolizumab pegol	1	1.6
Tocilizumab	1	1.6
Ixekizumab	4	6.3
Secukinumab	3	4.7
Guselkumab	1	1.6
Steroids	1	1.6
Apremilast	2	3.1
Ascorbic acid, calcium Pantothenate	2	3.1
Biotin	2	3.1

bDMARDs, biologic disease modifying antirheumatic drugs; csDMARDs, conventional synthetic disease modifying antirheumatic drugs; NSAIDs, nonsteroidal anti-inflammatory drugs.

Table 7.
The treatment status for psoriatic arthritis.

adalimumab and infliximab, which were both prescribed in 10 cases (15.6%), followed by ixekizumab in 4 cases (6.3%), etanercept and sekukinumab both in 3 cases (4.7%), and certolizumab pegol, tocilizumab, and guselkumab each prescribed in 1 case (1.6%). Other treatments included prednisolone in a single case (1.6%) and apremilast, ascorbic acid, calcium pantothenate, and biotin, each prescribed in two cases (3.1%) (**Table 7**).

4. Discussion

We identified several clinical features of PsA based on the results of this study. First, PsA dominantly afflicted male patients (77%), with the mean age of onset for cutaneous psoriasis at 36.8 years, while that of osteoarticular lesions at 47.0 years. Second, the skin leading type was observed more than the osteoarticular leading type, with the interval between the onset of both symptoms significantly shorter in the osteoarticular leading type than in the skin leading type. Third, upper extremity lesions were more dominant (53 cases; 83%) than lower extremity lesions (30 cases; 47%). Fourth, axial lesions were observed in 33% and enthesitis in 23% of the sample. Fifth, obesity was strongly associated with PsA. Finally, csDMARDs were the most prescribed drugs in patients with PsA, followed by bDMARDs and NSAIDs.

Regarding the onset pattern of PsA in a Japanese multicenter study, Ohara reported arthritis preceded psoriasis in 11% of patients [1]. In previous reports concerning PsA [3–6], the incidences of "joint before skin" cases were between 15% and 30% of the sample. In our study, arthritis preceded skin lesions in 17%, which was in near agreement with the results of previous reports. In these cases, the lack of skin lesions makes diagnosis difficult.

Regarding the distribution of arthritis, Ritchlin reported that axial joints are affected in 50% of PsA patients [2]. In the Japanese multicenter study, back pain such as lumbago and neck pain was observed in 34.3% of patients and enthesitis in 28.3% [10, 11]. Similarly, our study showed that axial lesions were present in 33% and enthesitis in 23%.

Moreover, we checked the distribution of arthritis by the onset patterns in this study. However, there was no statistically significant difference in both peripheral and axial lesions, and it was therefore concluded that the distribution pattern was not useful for detecting PsA in the osteoarticular leading type.

The risk factors for the development of psoriasis are obesity and lifestyle-related diseases such as hypertension, diabetes mellitus, hyperlipidemia [12], with obesity-related to the severity of psoriasis [13]. A large cohort study also demonstrated that BMI was associated with psoriasis [14]. In another study, PsA showed a significant association with obesity, type 2 diabetes, hypertension, metabolic syndrome, fatty liver, and an increased risk of cardiovascular events [15].

Similarly, in our study, obesity was significantly associated with PsA; however, the other factors were not statistically significantly associated with PsA.

Regarding the treatment status, NSAIDs were effective for joint symptoms but ineffective for skin lesions. The csDMARDs were effective for arthritis and skin involvement, whereas the bDMARDs were used for patients with an inadequate response to the csDMARDs as it can suppress skin and joint inflammation and delay radiographic progression.

Despite the use of traditional disease-modifying medications in more than 50% of patients with PsA, bone erosions were still observed in 47% of patients within the first 2 years [16]. Therefore, the appropriate diagnosis of PsA and tight control are required for better clinical outcomes of PsA. According to the American College of Rheumatology recommendation for PsA in a 2019 update, non-steroidal anti-inflammatory drugs and local glucocorticoid injections are proposed as initial therapy. Further, for patients with arthritis and poor prognostic factors such as polyarthritis or monoarthritis/oligoarthritis accompanied by factors such as dactylitis or joint damage, rapid initiation of csDMARDs are recommended. If the treatment target is not achieved with this strategy, bDMARDs targeting tumor necrosis factor (TNF), interleukin (IL)-17A, or IL-12/23 should be initiated [17].

In our study, NSAIDs were used in 39% of patients, csDMARDS in 64%, and bDMARDs in 51.5%. These data suggest that skin or arthritic symptoms were moderate to high in our cases. Yamamoto et al. Demonstrated that bDMARDs were used in more than 50% of all patients registered with PsA, which is in agreement with our results [10, 11].

Our study had several limitations. First, the small sample size was a result of this study taking place at a single center. Second, the type of skin and severity of psoriasis with a Psoriasis Area and Severity Index score was not evaluated. Third, the effect of the prescribed drugs was not examined.

5. Conclusions

we clarified the clinical features of PsA in a clinical orthopedic outpatient clinic setting. PsA was more dominant in male patients, with the osteoarticular leading type pattern of PsA observed in 17% of patients, as opposed to 75% in the skin leading type pattern. The interval between the onset of osteoarticular symptoms and the appearance of skin lesions was 4.5 years on average in the osteoarticular leading type, which was significantly shorter than that in the skin leading type. It was concluded that for patients with RF negative polyarthritis, it is important to be aware that psoriasis may develop approximately 4 years on average. Increased use of csDMARDs and bDMARDs was observed compared to that of NSAIDs.

Acknowledgements

The authors acknowledge English language editing and proofreading for Editage.

Conflicts of interest

None.

Ethical statement

This study was performed with the approval of the institutional review board of our hospital.

Author details

Naoki Kondo*, Masahiko Yamada and Rika Kakutani
Division of Orthopedic Surgery, Department of Orthopedic Surgery,
Niigata University Graduate School of Medical and Dental Sciences, Niigata, Japan

*Address all correspondence to: naokikondo1214@gmail.com

References

[1] Ohara Y, Kishimoto M, Takizawa N, et al. Prevalence and clinical characteristics of psoriatic arthritis in Japan. The Journal of Rheumatology. 2015;**42**:1439-1442

[2] Ritchlin CT, Colbert RA, Gladman DD. Psoriatic arthritis. The New England Journal of Medicine. 2017;**376**:2095-2096

[3] Gladman DD, Antoni C, Mease P, et al. Psoriatic arthritis: Epidemiology, clinical features, course, and outcome. Annals of the Rheumatic Diseases. 2005;**64**(Supplement 2):ii14-ii17

[4] Torre Alonso JC, Rodriguez Perez A, Arribas Castrillo JM, et al. Psoriatic arthritis (PA): A clinical, immunological and radiological study of 180 patients. British Journal of Rheumatology. 1991;**30**:245-250

[5] Gladman DD, Shuckett R, Russell ML, et al. Psoriatic arthritis (PSA)-an analysis of 220 patients. The Quarterly Journal of Medicine. 1987;**62**:127-141

[6] Kammer GM, Soter NA, Gibson DJ, et al. Psoriatic arthritis: A clinical, immunologic and HLA study of 100 patients. Seminars in Arthritis and Rheumatism. 1979;**9**:75-97

[7] Taylor W, Gladman D, Helliwell P, et al. Classification criteria for psoriatic arthritis: Development of new criteria from a large international study. Arthritis and Rheumatism. 2006;**54**:2665-2673

[8] Perez-Chada LM, Merola JF. Comorbidities associated with psoriatic arthritis: Review and update. Clinical Immunology. 2020;**214**:108397

[9] National Health and Nutrition Survey (Heisei 28 nen). Available from: https://www.mhlw.go.jp/stf/houdou/0000177189.html

[10] Yamamoto T, Kawada A. Clinical characteristics of Japanese patients with psoriatic arthritis: Comparison with East Asian countries. The Journal of Dermatology. 2018;**45**:273-278

[11] Yamamoto T, Ohtsuki M, Sano S, et al. Epidemiological analysis of psoriatic arthritis patients in Japan. The Journal of Dermatology. 2016;**43**:1193-1196

[12] Kamiya K, Kishimoto M, Sugai J, et al. Risk factors for the development of psoriasis. International Journal of Molecular Sciences. 2019;**20**:4347

[13] Tobin AM, Hackett CB, Rogers S, et al. Body mass index, waist circumference and HOMA-IR correlate with the Psoriasis Area and Severity Index in patients with psoriasis receiving phototherapy. The British Journal of Dermatology. 2014;**171**:436-438

[14] Setty AR, Curhan G, Choi HK. Obesity, waist circumference, weight change, and the risk of psoriasis in women: Nurses' Health Study II. Archives of Internal Medicine. 2007;**167**:1670-1675

[15] Ogdie A, Schwartzman S, Husni ME. Recognizing and managing comorbidities in psoriatic arthritis. Current Opinion in Rheumatology. 2015;**27**:118-126

[16] Kane D, Stafford L, Bresnihan B, et al. A prospective, clinical and radiological study of early psoriatic

arthritis: An early synovitis clinic experience. Rheumatology (Oxford). 2003;**42**:1460-1468

[17] Gossec L, Baraliakos X, Kerschbaumer A, et al. EULAR recommendations for the management of psoriatic arthritis with pharmacological therapies: 2019 update. Annals of the Rheumatic Diseases. 2020;**79**:700-712

Chapter 2

Dermoscopic Differential Diagnosis of Psoriasis

Ece Gokyayla, Tubanur Cetinarslan and Aylin Turel Ermertcan

Abstract

Psoriasis is a chronic inflammatory skin disease, which is mainly characterized with erythematous indurated plaques with squams such as many other inflammatory skin diseases. Also different clinical subtypes of psoriasis can show distinctive clinical appearances. As an example, inverse psoriasis does not have squams and resemble erythema intertrigo; or erythrodermic variant cannot be distinguished from other erythroderma causes sometimes. From reasons above, differential diagnosis of psoriasis should be done carefully to manage a chronic and long-term treatment required disease appropriately. Histopathologial examination is gold standard technique for certain diagnosis; however, dermoscope is a noninvasive and easily applicable diagnostic tool with high specificity. In this chapter, we discuss dermoscopic differential diagnosis of psoriasis.

Keywords: psoriasis, dermoscopy, inflammoscopy

1. Introduction

Psoriasis is a chronic inflammatory skin disease that progresses with remission and exacerbations [1, 2]. It constitutes an important percentage, approximately 6–8% of patients who apply to dermatology clinics [3]. Due to its high prevalence and chronic course, it is important to diagnose it early and clearly to manage patient appropriately and avoid functional losses as much as possible. In addition, in some situations that should be intervened swiftly such as erythrodermic psoriasis or generalized pustular psoriasis; the sooner we diagnose, the better we take control of disease setting.

In diagnosis of psoriasis, usually clinical observation is enough; however, in doubtful cases, histopathological examination is required as gold standard technique. However, it requires an invasive procedure and needs time for pathological preparation. With dermoscopy, we can mostly distinguish psoriasis from other resembling diseases in clinic noninvasively. Despite it not being gold standard, easily applicable and noninvasive properties of dermoscopy make it a helpful diagnostic tool and reduce the need of performing biopsies.

2. Dermoscopy of psoriasis types and differentials

2.1 Plaque psoriasis

Plaque psoriasis is the most common clinical subtype of psoriasis with 90% of all cases [4]. It is characterized by erythematous, well-defined, and usually indurated plaques greater than 1 cm in size with white-silvery scales on them (**Figure 1**). They can vary in size and may coalesce. Especially rapidly progressing lesions can be seen in annular configuration (**Figure 2**) [4, 5]. Removal of psoriatic scales may cause pin-point bleedings, which is called Auspitz sign. Psoriatic plaques are mostly located in the scalp, trunk, lumbosacral area, and extensor surfaces of extremities (**Figure 3**) [6].

2.1.1 Dermoscopy of plaque psoriasis

Dermoscopic examination of a psoriasis plaque should be done in three categories: background, vessels, and scales. Examination should be done with minimal pressure to visualize vessels better and with immersion oil if possible.

In dermoscopic examination of plaque psoriasis with handheld dermoscope, we usually see regularly distributed dotted vessels in a reddish-pinkish background and white scales (**Figure 4**) [7]. In some cases, background can be grayish-white due to highly hyperkeratotic scales (**Figure 5**).

Apart from regular distribution, vessels can be distributed scattered, in clusters, in rings, and patchy (**Figure 6a**). In higher magnifications (with videodermoscopy), these dotted vessels can be seen as bushy capillaries, globules, radial capillaries, globular rings, hairpin capillaries, and comma vessels in descending order [8] (**Figure 6b**). Rarely dot blood hemorrhages can be seen in vessel locations (**Figure 5**). Scales can be distributed diffuse, patchy, central, or peripheral in descending order; however, white color is key point for scales [8, 9].

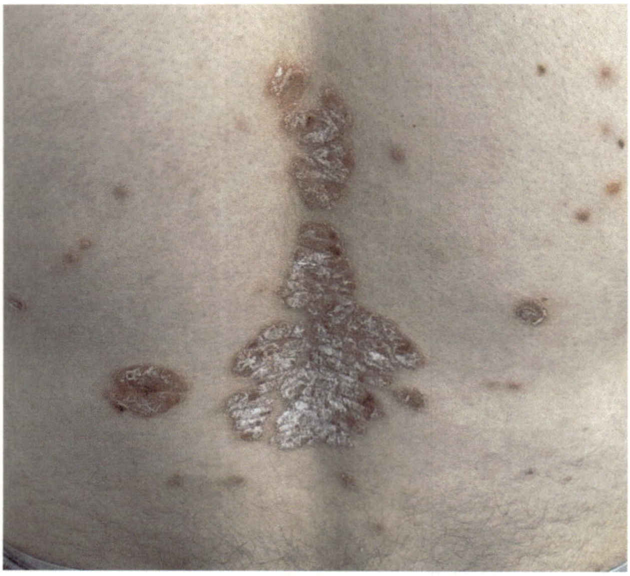

Figure 1.
Erythematous, well-defined indurated plaque with white scales.

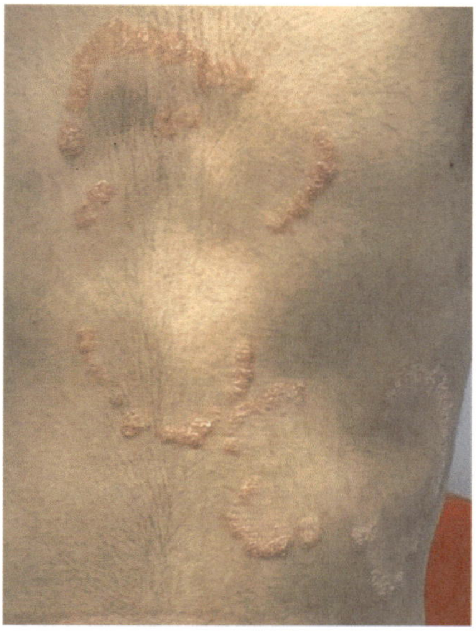

Figure 2.
Erythematous, annular plaques with white scales.

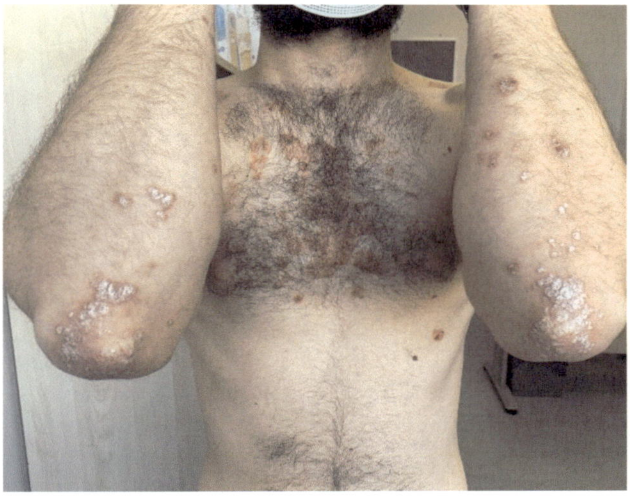

Figure 3.
Psoriatic plaques located on the trunk and extensor surfaces of the arms.

2.1.2 Dermoscopic differential diagnosis of plaque psoriasis

Differential diagnosis of plaque psoriasis should be done with skin diseases, which are characterized by erythematous plaques with scales such as dermatitis, tinea corporis, pityriasis rosea, pityriasis rubra pilaris, lichen planus, and non-pigmented squamous cell carcinoma in situ.

In dermoscopic examination of dermatitis, we usually see patchy or scattered distributed dotted vessels with yellow globules (corresponding to sero-crusts) [10]. Background can be erythematous or not depending on lesions phase (acute or

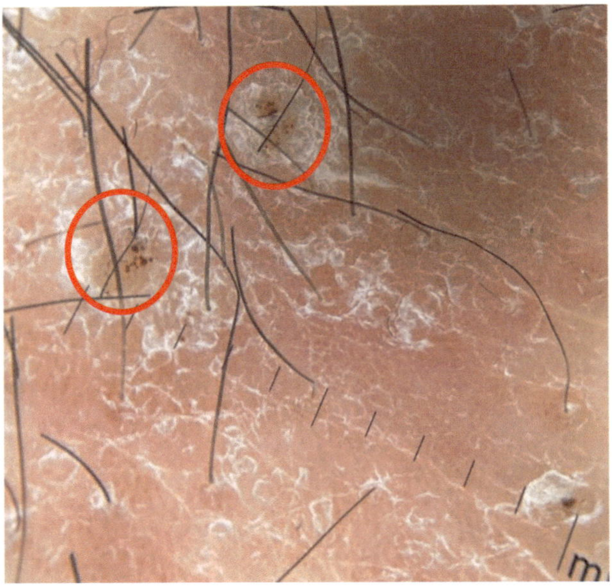

Figure 4.
Regularly distributed dotted vessels on reddish background with patchy distributed white scales. Note dot blood hemorrhages (red circle). Anatomical localization: Upper extremity (×10).

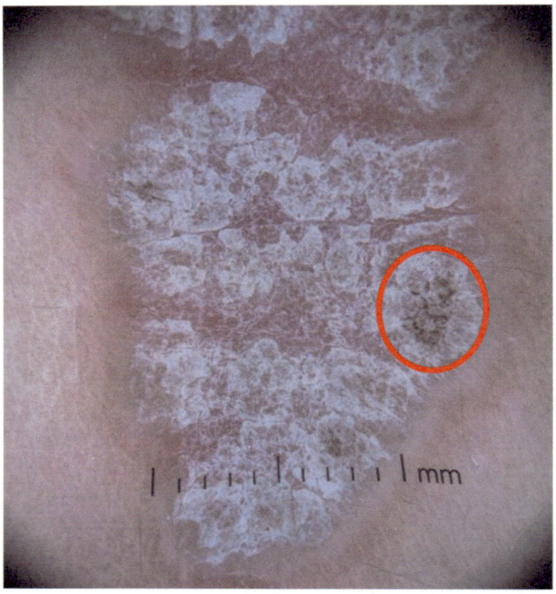

Figure 5.
Background color can barely be seen due to diffuse thick white scales. Dotted vessels can be seen in the center. Note dot blood hemorrhages (red circle). Anatomical localization: Elbow (×10).

chronic). Hemorrhagic crusts can be seen as well secondary to traumatization (**Figure 7**).

In dermoscopic examination of tinea corporis, we usually see peripherally located dotted vessels and rough white scales (**Figure 8**). In contrast with psoriasis, dotted

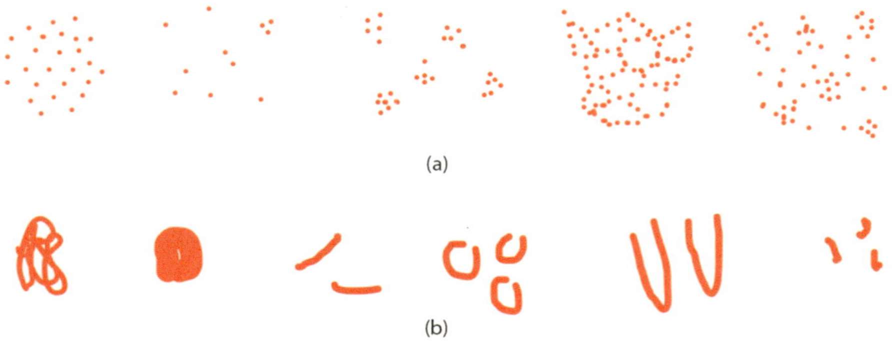

Figure 6.
a: Vessel distribution patterns (regular, scattered, in clusters, in rings, patchy, respectively). b: Vessels subtypes can be seen in higher magnifications (bushy, globular, radial, globular ring, hairpin, and comma vessels, respectively).

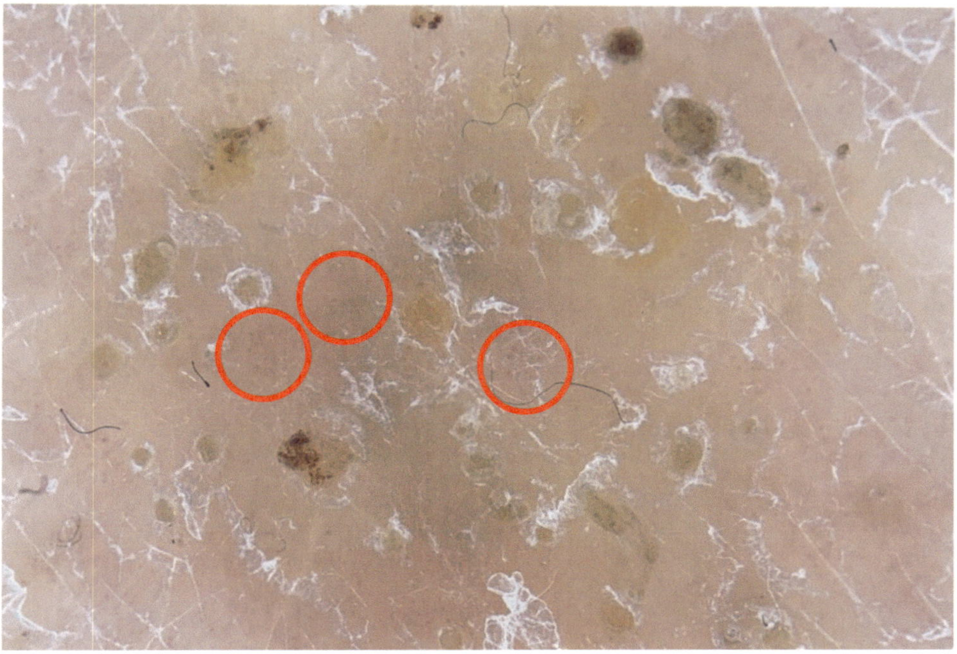

Figure 7.
Yellow globules, dot blood hemorrhages, and hemorrhagic crusts, patchy distributed dotted vessels (red circle). Background is slightly pinkish. Anatomical localization: Lower extremity (×20).

vessels are not regularly distributed and not uniform. In addition, scales are only located peripherally, tend to peel outward, and shaped in moth-eaten pattern [11].

Pityriasis rubra pilaris shows dotted and more frequently linear vessels, perifollicular yellow-orange halos, follicular plugs with central hair on them (**Figure 9**). Scales can be yellowish or whitish. Background is usually dark or yellowish red [7, 12].

Squamous cell carcinoma in situ and psoriasis can be challenging especially in solitary plaques. Dermoscopic clues for non-pigmented squamous cell carcinoma in situ are dotted or glomerular vessels in clusters in the center and arranged in lines at the periphery with yellowish white scales (**Figure 10**) [13, 14].

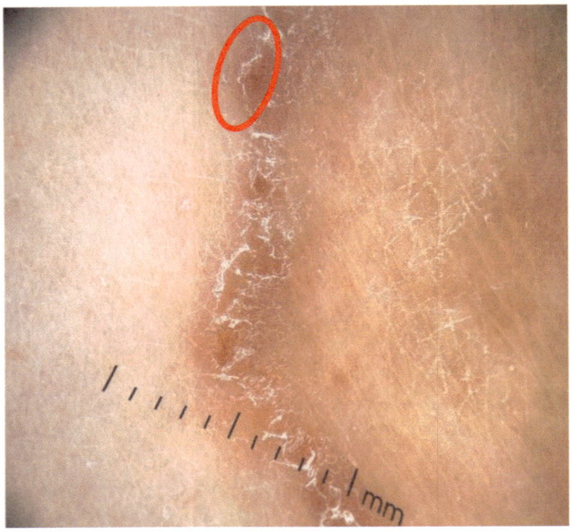

Figure 8.
Peripherally located dotted vessels and white scales. Note the moth-eaten pattern (red circle). Anatomical localization: Trunk (×10).

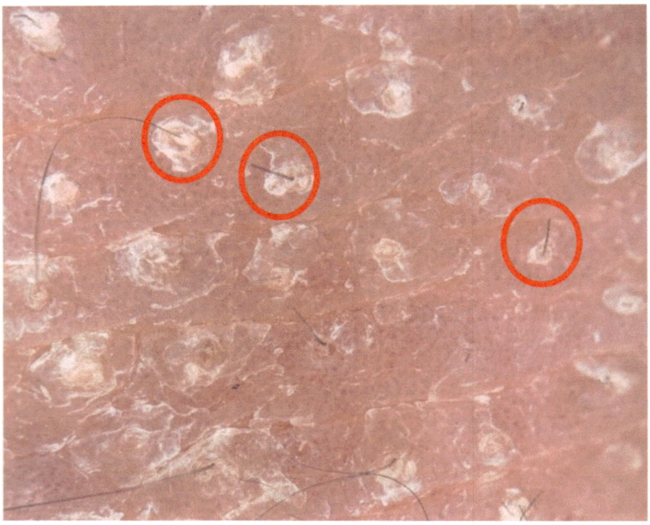

Figure 9.
Dotted vessels regularly distributed on pinkish background. Note the follicular plugs and central hairs (red circles). Anatomical localization: Elbow (×20).

Dermoscopic features of plaque psoriasis and its differentials are summarized in **Table 1**.

2.2 Guttate psoriasis

Guttate psoriasis, a psoriasis variant that is more common in pediatric population and young adults. Distinctly from other variants, we know that guttate psoriasis is selectively triggered by beta hemolytic streptococcal infections [15]. It is characterized by erythematous, well-defined flat papules/plaques lower than 1 cm in size with

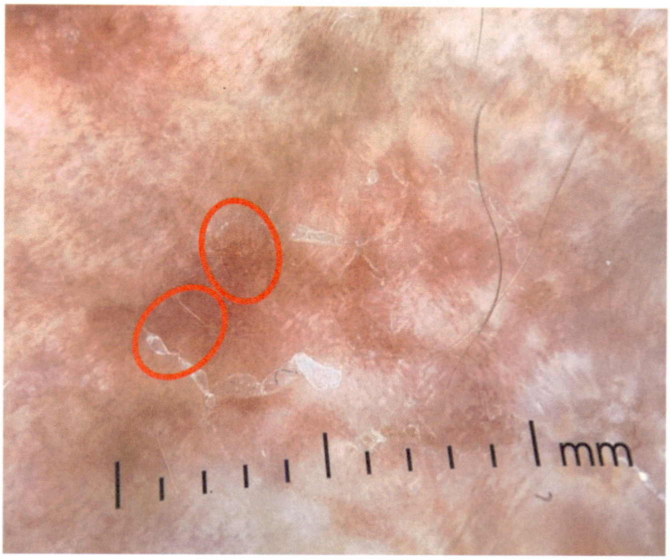

Figure 10.
Glomerular vessels in the center, white scales. Note the linear arrangement of dotted vessels at the periphery (red circles) and actinic keratosis area at top left. Anatomical localization: Forearm (×20).

	Background	Vessel types	Vessel arrangement	Scales	Additional features
Plaque psoriasis	Reddish-pinkish Whitish (due to hyperkeratotic scales)	Dotted	Regular	Whitish-grayish	
Dermatitis	Skin colored-pinkish	Dotted	Scattered/ patchy	Yellowish	Irregularly distributed dot blood hemorrhages due to traumatization
Tinea corporis	Reddish	Dotted	Peripheral	White and rough; peripheral; moth-eaten pattern; tend to peel outwards	
Pityriasis rubra pilaris	Dark red/ yellowish red	Linear and/ or dotted	Scattered	Yellowish-whitish; follicular	Perifollicular yellow-orange halos, follicular plugs, central hair
Squamous cell carcinoma in situ	Pinkish	Glomerular or dotted	Regularly in center, may organize in lines at the periphery	Yellowish white scales	Peripheral actinic keratosis areas may help (white and wide follicular openings, rosettes)

Table 1.
Dermoscopic features of plaque psoriasis and its differentials.

white-silvery scales on them. Lesions mostly located in the trunk and extremities (**Figure 11a** and **b**).

2.2.1 Dermoscopy of guttate psoriasis

Dermoscopic features of guttate psoriasis are very similar with plaque psoriasis, which is characterized by regularly distributed dotted vessels in a reddish background and white scales on them (**Figure 12**). Due to guttate psoriasis' smaller lesion sizes (lower than 1 cm in diameter), findings may be insignificant when compared with plaque psoriasis (**Figure 13**).

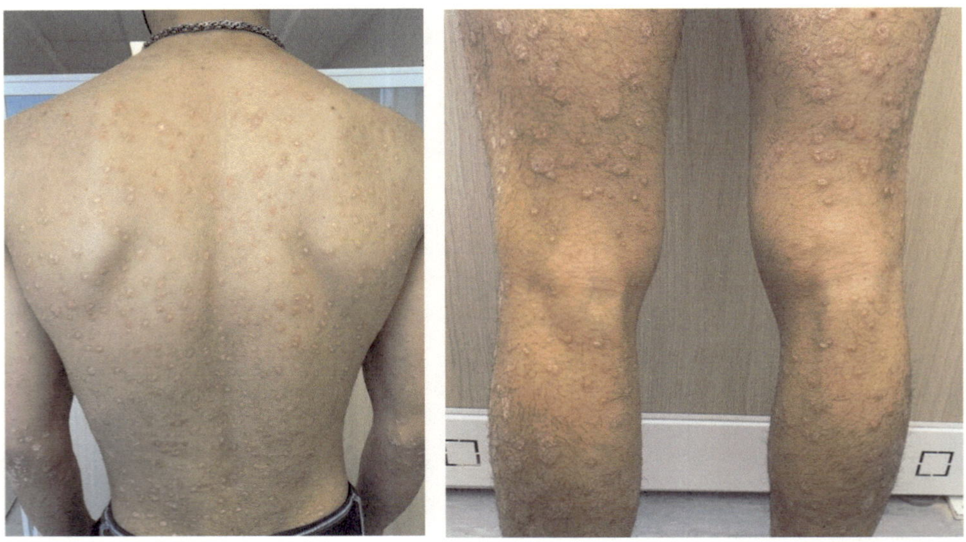

(a) (b)

Figure 11.
a: Slightly erythematous flat papules/plaques with white scales on them in an adolescent. Trunk localization. b: Slightly erythematous flat papules/plaques with white scales on them in an adolescent. Extremity localization.

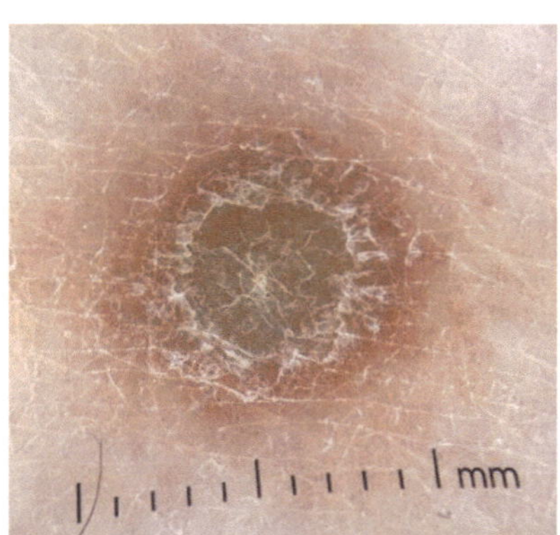

Figure 12.
Regularly distributed dotted vessels in reddish background. White scales. Anatomical localization: Upper extremity (×10).

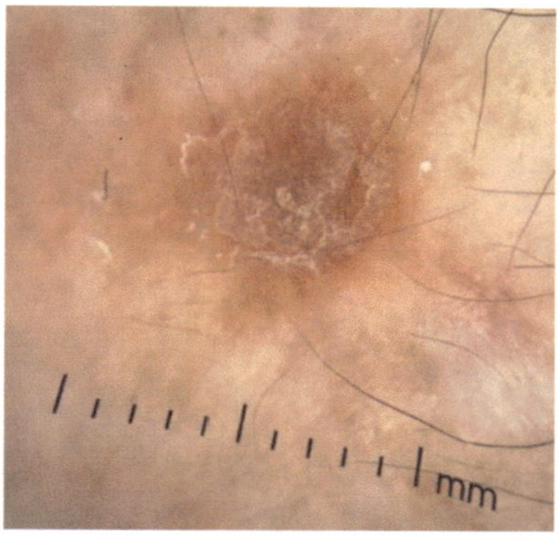

Figure 13.
Regularly distributed dotted vessels on pinkish background. Scales are white, thin, and patchy. Anatomical localization: Upper extremity (×10).

2.2.2 Dermoscopic differential diagnosis of guttate psoriasis

Differential diagnosis of guttate psoriasis should be done with skin diseases, which are characterized by erythematous papules/small plaques with scales. Pityriasis rosea, lichen planus, nummular dermatitis, secondary syphilis, tinea corporis, pityriasis lichenoides chronica, and disseminated eruptive porokeratosis may count as differential. (Dermatitis and tinea corporis will not be mentioned because they were discussed above.)

Dermoscopic examination of pityriasis rosea shows irregular distributed dotted vessels and peripheral thin white scale (**Figure 14**) [10]. Scales tend to peel outward as in tinea corporis. But note the white scale is not rough and vessels are not in the same distribution with scales. Background is generally skin-colored or slightly pinkish.

In dermoscopic examination of lichen planus, key point is detecting Wichkam striaes, which cannot be seen macroscopically sometimes. In fair-skinned patients,

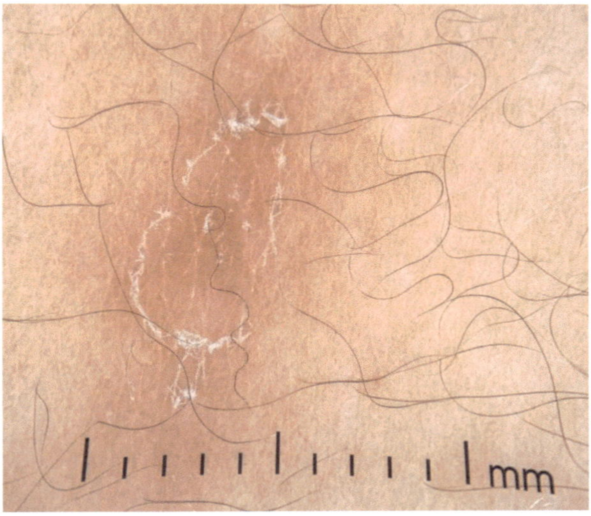

Figure 14.
Patchy distributed dotted vessels and peripheral thin white scale. The configuration of the scales named "collarette sign." anatomical localization: Back (×10).

dotted and linear vessels around Wickham striae make these structures more visible (**Figure 15**); however, in dark-skinned patients, absence of peripheral vascular structures around Wichkam striaes may lead to misdiagnosis [16].

In dermoscopic examination of secondary syphilis, yellowish-orange background and absence of vascular structures are key points (**Figure 16**) [17]. Scales may be present, however, thinner and smaller when compared with psoriatic scales.

In dermoscopic examination of pityriasis lichenoides chronica, we usually see orange-yellowish structureless areas and focally distributed dotted or linear vessels (**Figure 17**) [18].

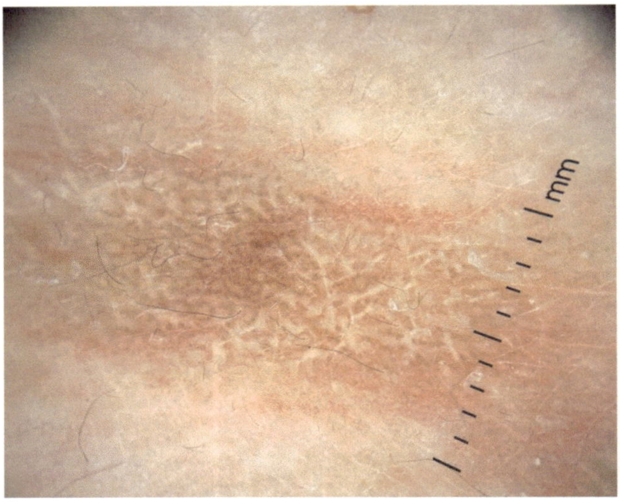

Figure 15.
Reticular arranged white lines (Wickham striae). Note the dotted vessels around Wickham striae in this fair-skinned patient. Anatomical localization: Lower extremity (×10).

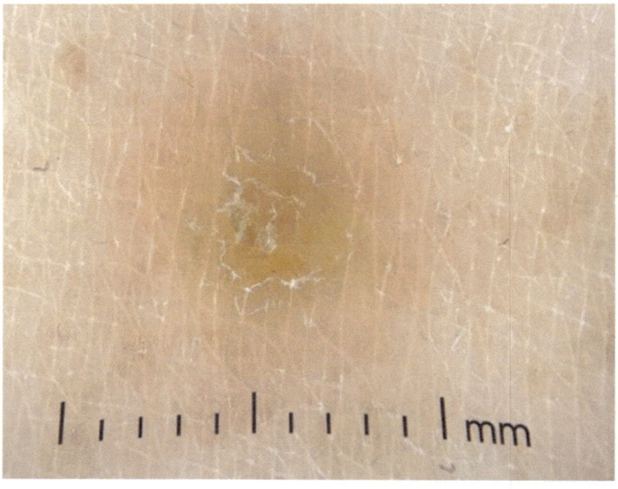

Figure 16.
Yellowish-orange structureless area with thin white scales. Note the absence of vascular structures. Anatomical localization: Back (×10).

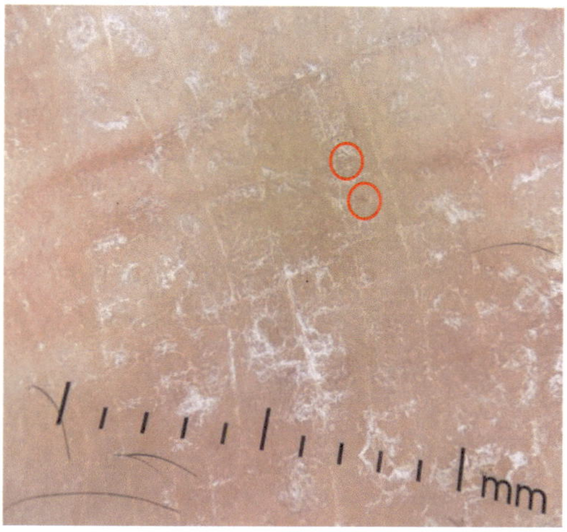

Figure 17.
Yellowish-orange structureless areas with thin white scales. Note the focal dotted vessel areas (red circles). Anatomical localization: Hand dorsum (×10).

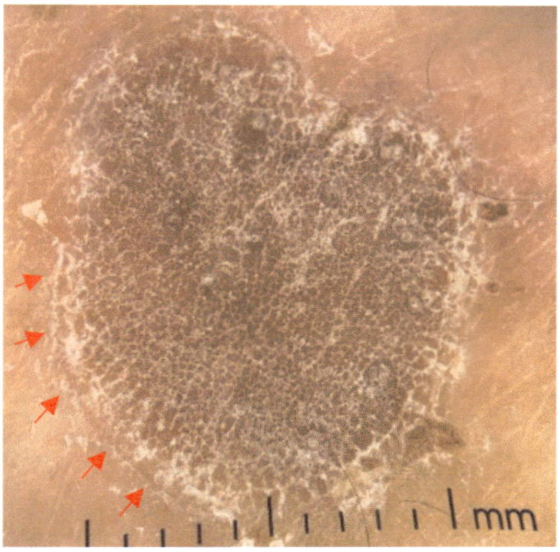

Figure 18.
Small white scales on yellowish-brown background. Note the railway-like "cornoid lamella" at the periphery (red arrows). Anatomical localization: Hand dorsum (×10).

In dermoscopic examination of porokeratosis, key clue is peripheral double lines resembling railways (**Figure 18**). This feature is called "cornoid lamella" [19].

Dermoscopic features of guttate psoriasis and its differentials are summarized in **Table 2**.

2.3 Inverse psoriasis

Inverse psoriasis is another clinical variant of psoriasis, which involves flexural areas such as axillary, inguinal, and inframammary [20]. The prevalence of inverse psoriasis is not clear and varies in 3–36% because of diagnostic challenges [21]. And also it is controversial that if genital involvement is a part of inverse psoriasis; however, we include genital involvement under this topic for convenience of expression.

	Background	Vessel types	Vessel arrangement	Scales	Additional features
Guttate psoriasis	Reddish-pinkish	Dotted	Regular	Whitish-grayish, thin and small	
Pityriasis rosea	Pinkish	Dotted (vascularization is not dominant)	Patchy	White, thin, peripheral and tend to peel outwards "collarette sign"	
Lichen planus	Pinkish, violaceus	Dotted or absent	Aroud Wickham striae	Whitish, patchy distributed, thin and small	
Secondary Syphilis	Yellowish-orange	Absent		White and thin	
Pityriasis lichenoides chronica	Pinkish, yellowish-orange	Dotted or linear	Focal	White, patchy, thin	
Disseminated porokeratosis	Yellowish-brown	Unsignificant		White, small	Peripheral railway like double lines called "cornoid lamella"

Table 2.
Dermoscopic features of guttate psoriasis and its differentials.

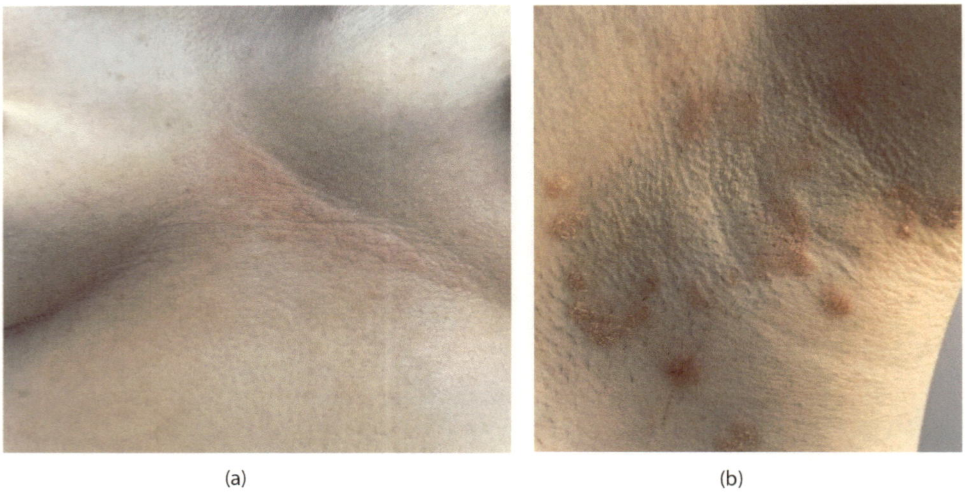

Figure 19.
a: Erythematous plaque located in inframammary fold. b: Erythematous papules and plaques located in axillary fold. Note peripheral lesions have mild white scales.

Inverse psoriasis is typically present with well-defined erythematous plaques located in flexural areas (**Figure 19a** and **b**). It can present with or without typical psoriasis plaques. In contrast with plaque and guttate psoriasis, scales are insignificant or absent.

Genital involvement shares similar clinical features with inverse psoriasis such as well-defined erythematous papules and plaques (**Figure 20**). However, occlusion in the genital areas is not as much as flexural areas, scales could be more visible in the genitals.

2.3.1 Dermoscopy of inverse psoriasis

Dermoscopic features of inverse psoriasis are characterized by regularly distributed dotted vessels on reddish background (**Figure 21**). In contrast with other variants, scales are absent. Absence of scales enhances visualization of vascular structures. Consequently, dermoscopic differential diagnosis of flexural dermatosis mainly leans on evaluation of vascular structures.

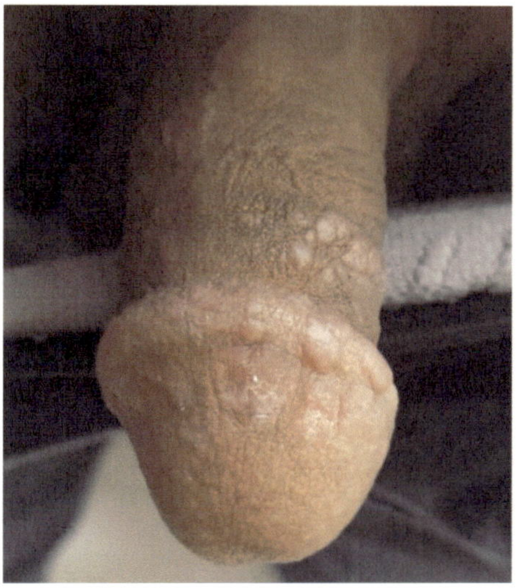

Figure 20.
Coalesced erythematous papules located in the glans penis and penile dorsum.

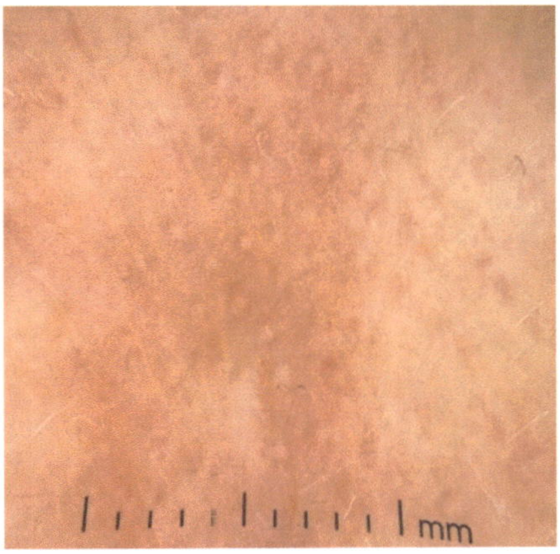

Figure 21.
Regularly distributed dotted vessels on pinkish background. Anatomical localization: Inframammary (×10).

2.3.2 Dermoscopic differential diagnosis of inverse psoriasis

Differential diagnosis of inverse psoriasis should be done with skin diseases, which present with erythematous patches/plaques in flexural and genital areas. Mechanical intertrigo, seborrheic dermatitis, lichen planus inversus, and fungal/bacterial infections may count as differential. Because no clear dermoscopic features have been defined for mechanical intertrigo and flexural infections, we will discuss dermoscopic features of seborrheic dermatitis and lichen planus inversus under this topic.

The main dermoscopic features of seborrheic dermatitis of flexural areas are irregularly distributed linear, blurry vessels [22]. As we mentioned before, we do not see classical yellowish scales of seborrheic dermatitis in flexuras.

When we review the literature so far, there are only three reports about dermoscopic features of lichen planus inversus. In all of these reports, dermoscopic features of only pigmented variant of lichen planus inversus were evaluated and defined as diffuse brown patches containing multiple granular gray-brown dots [23–25]. In our clinical practice, we see non-pigmented lichen planus inversus more than pigmented subtype. According to our dermoscopic experience, Wickham striae, which is seen in lichen planus inversus, tends to be in "starry sky" or "radial streaming" pattern rather than reticular pattern. Background is usually pinkish or violaceous. Dotted vessels usually encircle Wickham striae (**Figure 22**).

Dermoscopic features of inverse psoriasis and its differentials are summarized in **Table 3**.

2.4 Pustular psoriasis

Pustular psoriasis is a rare clinical variant of psoriasis, which is characterized by sterile pustules on an erythematous skin (**Figure 23**). It could be either local or generalized [26]. In generalized pustular psoriasis, concomitant fever, malaise, dehydration may also be present [27].

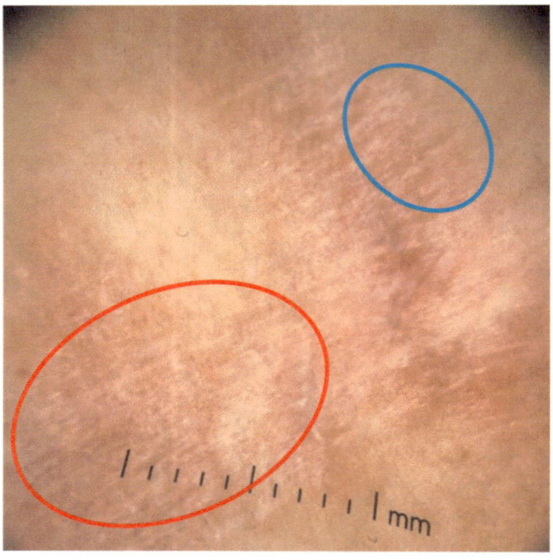

Figure 22.
Wickham striae in "radial streaming" pattern (red circle) and "starry sky" pattern (blue circle). Dotted vessels surround Wickham striae in a patchy arrangement. Anatomical localization: Intermammary (×10).

	Background	Vessel types	Vessel arrangement	Additional features
Inverse psoriasis	Reddish-pinkish	Dotted	Regular	
Seborrheic dermatitis of flexural areas	Pinkish	Linear, blurry vessels	Irregular	
Lichen planus inversus	Pinkish, violaceus	Dotted or absent	Aroud Wickham striae	According to our dermoscopic experience, Wickham striae, which is seen in lichen planus inversus, tends to be in "starry sky" or "radial streaming" pattern

Table 3.
Dermoscopic features of inverse psoriasis and its differentials.

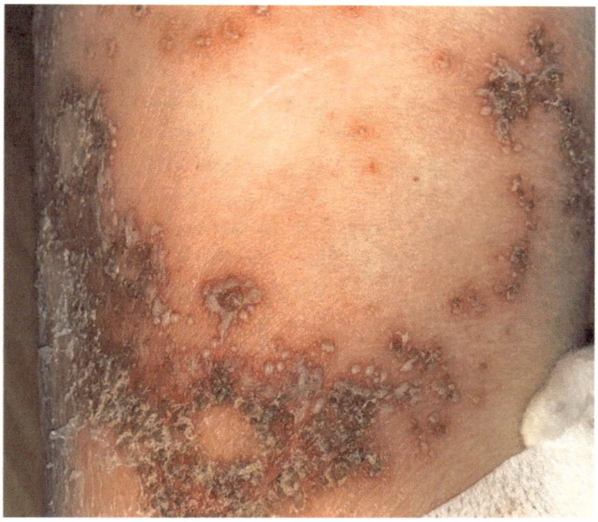

Figure 23.
Small pustules and lake of pus on erythematous background.

2.4.1 Dermoscopy of pustular psoriasis

Dermoscopic features of pustular psoriasis are characterized by regularly distributed dotted vessels with milky globules (corresponding to sterile pustules) on reddish background (**Figure 24**) [28]. Attention should be paid on non-follicular localization of pustules. Typical vascular structures are seen. Nonspecific yellow crust may be seen. Dermoscopic features are same in both localized and generalized subtypes.

2.4.2 Dermoscopic differential diagnosis of pustular psoriasis

Dermoscopic differential diagnosis of pustular psoriasis should be done with acute generalized exanthematous pustulosis (AGEP). In life-threatening clinical conditions such as generalized pustular eruptions, rapid and right diagnosis is essential, and dermoscope is very helpful at that point. In both pustular psoriasis and AGEP,

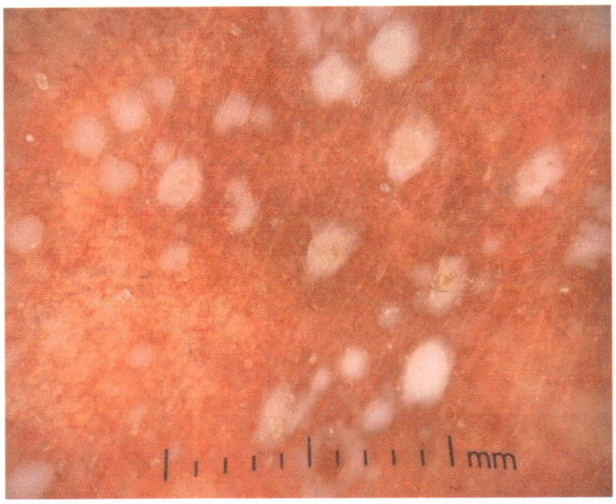

Figure 24.
Milky globules and regularly distributed dotted and bushy vessels on reddish background in pustular psoriasis. Anatomical localization: Trunk (×10).

pustules are sterile, disseminated, may coalesce, and be non-follicular. Thereby, we cannot distinguish these two situations by their clinical view only. In dermoscopic examination of both pustular psoriasis and AGEP, non-follicular milky globules on reddish background are seen [28]. Discriminately, in pustular psoriasis we see regularly distributed dotted vessels (**Figure 24**). In dermoscopic examination of AGEP, background is usually pinkish and vascular structures are absent (**Figure 25**) [29].

2.5 Erythrodermic psoriasis

Erythroderma is a life-threatening condition, which is defined as desquamation and erythema of more than 90% of body surface area [30]. Erythrodermic variant of psoriasis (**Figure 26**) generally occurs due to poor control of disease, withdrawal of anti-psoriatic treatments, triggering drug intake, underlying systemic infections or

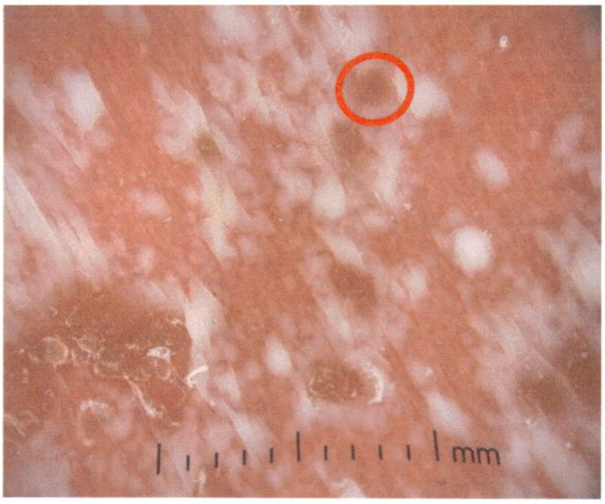

Figure 25.
Milky globules on reddish background. Globules are non-follicular (red circle). Note the absence of vessels. Anatomical localization: Trunk (×10).

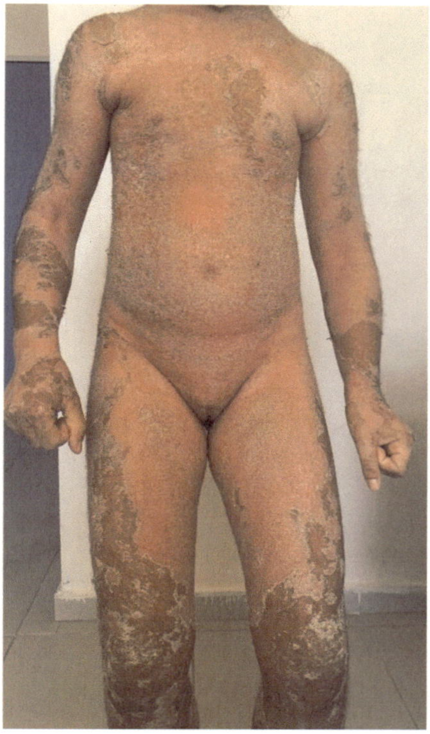

Figure 26.
Desquamation and erythema of all body surfaces.

conditions [31]. Clinical clues for erythrodermic psoriasis diagnosis are known history of psoriasis, psoriatic nail changes, presence of psoriatic arthritis. However, if none of the mentioned features is present, dermoscopy could be a game-changer.

2.5.1 Dermoscopy of erythrodermic psoriasis

Dermoscopic features of erythrodermic psoriasis are the same as other psoriasis variants. Regularly distributed dotted vessels on a reddish background, and patchy white scales are seen (**Figure 27**) [32].

2.5.2 Dermoscopic differential diagnosis of erythrodermic psoriasis

Dermoscopic differential diagnosis of erythrodermic psoriasis includes dermatosis that can present with erythroderma such as atopic dermatitis, mycosis fungoides, and pityriasis rubra pilaris (Pityriasis rubra pilaris will not be mentioned because it was discussed above.)

Dermoscopic examination of atopic dermatitis shows typical dermatitis features. Yellowish globules (corresponding to sero-crusts) and patchy distributed dotted vessels on a pinkish background are demonstrative (**Figure 28**) [32].

Dermoscopic features of erythrodermic mycosis fungoides are a combination of linear and dotted vessels on a pale pinkish background (**Figure 29**) [32]. Some short linear vessels may be curved and named as "spermatozoon-like" vessels.

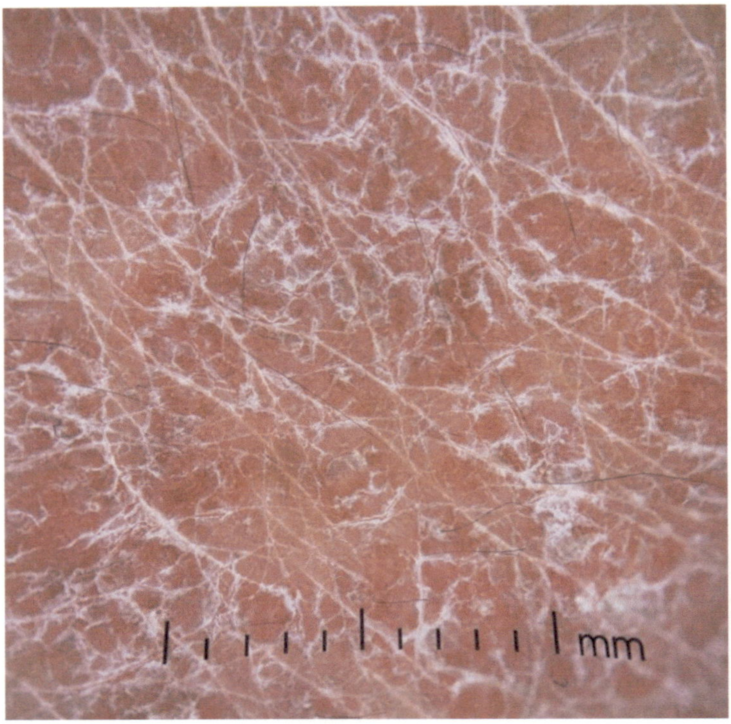

Figure 27.
Regularly distributed dotted vessels and white scales. Anatomical localization: Lower extremity (×20).

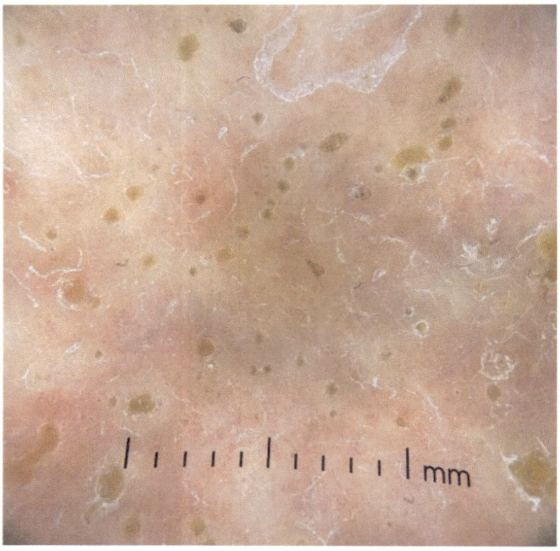

Figure 28.
Yellow globules, patchy distributed dotted vessels. Background is slightly pinkish. Tiny white scales are also present. Tiny white scales correspond to desquamation areas. Anatomical localization: Trunk (×10).

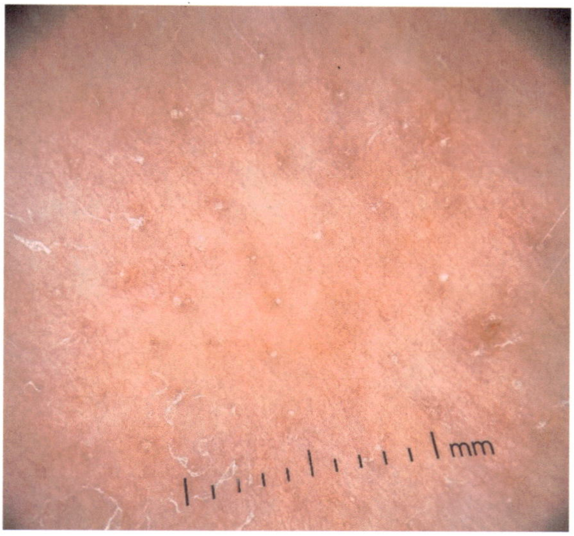

Figure 29.
Linear, serpiginous, and dotted vessels on pinkish background. Tiny white scales correspond to desquamation areas. Anatomical localization: Trunk (×10).

	Background	Vessel types	Vessel arrangement	Scales	Additional features
Erythrodermic psoriasis	Reddish	Dotted	Regular	White, scattered-patchy scales	
Erythrodermic atopic dermatitis	Pinkish	Dotted	Patchy	Yellowish sero-crusts	
Erythrodermic mycosis fungoides	Pinkish (pale)	Linear and dotted	Scattered	Whitish scales can present.	.

Table 4.
Dermoscopic features of erythrodermic psoriasis and its differentials.

Dermoscopic features of erythrodermic psoriasis and its differentials are summarized in **Table 4**.

3. Conclusions

Psoriasis is a common skin disease with different clinical presentations. Generally, clinical evaluation is enough for diagnosis, though dermoscope is a helpful and noninvasive examination technique that enhances true diagnosis ratio. Knowing psoriasis' and its differentials' dermoscopic features may reduce requirement for histopathological examination and also makes rapid diagnosis possible in life-threatening conditions such as erythroderma. Note that regularly distributed dotted vessels on a reddish background are the most important clues for any variant of psoriasis. In doubtful cases, histopathological examination should be done for verifying the diagnosis as a gold standard technique.

Acknowledgements

All photos used in this chapter were taken by Dr. Ece Gokyayla with iPhone (XS) and dermatoscope (DermLite, DL4 model, 3Gen, USA) connected to an iPhone (XS) via adapter (DermLite Connection Kit MagnetiConnect). Immersion oil was not used. *Written informed* consent will be obtained from each patient in *oral and written* form. Only histopathologically or laboratorially confirmed cases' photographs were included.

Conflict of interest

The authors declare no conflict of interest and no funding source.

Author details

Ece Gokyayla[1], Tubanur Cetinarslan[2] and Aylin Turel Ermertcan[1]*

1 Medical Faculty, Department of Dermatology and Venereology, Manisa Celal Bayar University, Manisa, Turkey

2 Department of Dermatology and Venereology, Kirikkale Training Hospital, Kirikkale, Turkey

*Address all correspondence to: draylinturel@hotmail.com

References

[1] Gül Ü. Psoriasis. Sağlığın Başkenti Dergisi. 2010;**16**:18-21

[2] Griffiths CEM, Camp RDR, Barker JNWN. Psoriasis. In: Burns T, Breathnach S, Cox N, Griffiths C, editors. Rook's Textbook of Dermatology. 7th ed. Oxford: Blackwell; 2004. pp. 35.1-35.69

[3] Braun-Falco O, Plewig G, Wolff HH, Burgdorf WHC. Dermatology. 2nd ed. Berlin: Springer-Verlag Berlin Heidelberg; 2000. pp. 585-610

[4] Griffiths CE, Barker JN. Pathogenesis and clinical features of psoriasis. Lancet. 2007;**370**(9583):263-271. DOI: 10.1016/S0140-6736(07)61128-3

[5] Langley RG, Krueger GG, Griffiths CE. Psoriasis: Epidemiology, clinical features, and quality of life. Annals of the Rheumatic Diseases. 2005;**64**(Suppl 2):ii18-ii23; discussion ii24-5. DOI: 10.1136/ard.2004.033217

[6] Weigle N, McBane S. Psoriasis. American Family Physician. 2013;**87**(9):626-633

[7] Jha AK, Lallas A, Sonthalia S, Jhakar D, Udayan UK, Chaudhary RKP. Differentiation of pityriasis rubra pilaris from plaque psoriasis by dermoscopy. Dermatology Practical & Conceptual. 2018;**8**(4):299-302. DOI: 10.5826/dpc.0804a10

[8] Golińska J, Sar-Pomian M, Rudnicka L. Dermoscopic features of psoriasis of the skin, scalp and nails - A systematic review. Journal of the European Academy of Dermatology and Venereology. 2019;**33**(4):648-660. DOI: 10.1111/jdv.15344

[9] Golińska J, Sar-Pomian M, Rudnicka L. Dermoscopy of plaque psoriasis differs with plaque location, its duration, and patient's sex. Skin Research and Technology. 2021;**27**(2):217-226. DOI: 10.1111/srt.12933

[10] Errichetti E, Stinco G. Dermoscopy in general dermatology: A practical overview. Dermatology and Therapy. 2016;**6**(4):471-507. DOI: 10.1007/s13555-016-0141-6

[11] Lekkas D, Ioannides D, Lazaridou E, Lallas A, Apalla Z, Vakirlis E, et al. Dermatoscopy of tinea corporis. Journal of the European Academy of Dermatology and Venereology. 2020;**34**(6):e278-e280. DOI: 10.1111/jdv.16277

[12] Abdel-Azim NE, Ismail SA, Fathy E. Differentiation of pityriasis rubra pilaris from plaque psoriasis by dermoscopy. Archives of Dermatological Research. 2017;**309**:311-314

[13] Wozniak-Rito AM, Rudnicka L. Bowen's disease in Dermoscopy. Acta Dermatovenerologica Croatica. 2018;**26**(2):157-161

[14] Zalaudek I, Argenziano G. Dermoscopy of actinic keratosis, intraepidermal carcinoma and squamous cell carcinoma. Current Problems in Dermatology. 2015;**46**:70-76. DOI: 10.1159/000366539

[15] Saleh D, Tanner LS. Guttate Psoriasis. In: StatPearls. Treasure Island (FL): StatPearls Publishing; 2021

[16] García-García B, Munguía-Calzada P, Aubán-Pariente J, Argenziano G, Vázquez-López F. Dermoscopy of lichen planus: Vascular and Wickham striae variations in the skin of colour. The Australasian Journal of Dermatology. 2019;**60**(4):301-304. DOI: 10.1111/ajd.13052

[17] Mathur M, Acharya P, Karki A, Shah J, Kc N. Dermoscopic clues in the skin lesions of secondary syphilis. Clinical Case Reports. 2019;**7**(3): 431-434. DOI: 10.1002/ccr3.1999

[18] Errichetti E, Lacarrubba F, Micali G, Piccirillo A, Stinco G. Differentiation of pityriasis lichenoides chronica from guttate psoriasis by dermoscopy. Clinical and Experimental Dermatology. 2015; **40**(7):804-806. DOI: 10.1111/ced.12580

[19] Idoudi S, Dalle S. Dermoscopie de la porokératose actinique disséminée superficielle [Dermoscopy of disseminated superficial actinic porokeratosis]. Annales de Dermatologie et de Vénéréologie. 2020;**147**(12): 914-915. French. DOI: 10.1016/j.annder.2020.05.003

[20] Micali G, Verzì AE, Giuffrida G, Panebianco E, Musumeci ML, Lacarrubba F. Inverse psoriasis: From diagnosis to current treatment options. Clinical, Cosmetic and Investigational Dermatology. 2019;**12**:953-959. DOI: 10.2147/CCID.S189000

[21] Omland SH, Gniadecki R. Psoriasis inversa: A separate identity or a variant of psoriasis vulgaris? Clinics in Dermatology. 2015;**33**(4):456-461. DOI: 10.1016/j.clindermatol.2015.04.007

[22] Errichetti E, Lacarrubba F, Micali G, Stinco G. Dermoscopy of Zoon's plasma cell balanitis. Journal of the European Academy of Dermatology and Venereology. 2016;**30**(12):e209-e210. DOI: 10.1111/jdv.13538

[23] Robles-Méndez JC, Rizo-Frías P, Herz-Ruelas ME, Pandya AG, Ocampo CJ. Lichen planus pigmentosus and its variants: Review and update. International Journal of Dermatology. 2018;**57**(5):505-514. DOI: 10.1111/ijd.13806

[24] Imbernón-Moya A, Churruca-Grijelmo M, Martínez-Pérez M, Lobato-Berezo A. Dermoscopic features of lichen planus Pigmentosus-Inversus. Actas Dermo-Sifiliográficas. 2015; **106**(10):857-859. English, Spanish. DOI: 10.1016/j.ad.2015.06.007

[25] Murzaku EC, Bronsnick T, Rao BK. Axillary lichen planus pigmentosus-inversus: Dermoscopic clues of a rare entity. Diagnosis: Lichen planus pigmentosus (LPP). Journal of the American Academy of Dermatology. 2014;**71**(4):e119-e120. DOI: 10.1016/j.jaad.2014.01.881

[26] Hoegler KM, John AM, Handler MZ, Schwartz RA. Generalized pustular psoriasis: A review and update on treatment. Journal of the European Academy of Dermatology and Venereology. 2018;**32**(10):1645-1651. DOI: 10.1111/jdv.14949

[27] Bachelez H. Pustular psoriasis and related pustular skin diseases. The British Journal of Dermatology. 2018;**178**(3):614-618. DOI: 10.1111/bjd.16232

[28] Errichetti E, Stinco G. Dermatoscopy in life-threatening and severe acute rashes. Clinics in Dermatology. 2020; **38**(1):113-121. DOI: 10.1016/j.clindermatol.2019.10.013

[29] Jha AK, Sonthalia S, Lallas A. Non-follicular milky globules-dermoscopy saves the day. Dermatology Practical & Conceptual. 2017;**7**(2):35-36. DOI: 10.5826/dpc.0702a07

[30] Cuellar-Barboza A, Ocampo-Candiani J, Herz-Ruelas ME. A practical approach to the diagnosis and treatment of adult erythroderma. Actas Dermosifiliogr. 2018;**109**(9):777-790. DOI: 10.1016/j.ad.2018.05.011

[31] Raychaudhuri SK, Maverakis E, Raychaudhuri SP. Diagnosis and classification of psoriasis. Autoimmunity Reviews. 2014;**13**(4–5):490-495. DOI: 10.1016/j.autrev.2014.01.008

[32] Errichetti E, Piccirillo A, Stinco G. Dermoscopy as an auxiliary tool in the differentiation of the main types of erythroderma due to dermatological disorders. International Journal of Dermatology. 2016;**55**(12):e616-e618. DOI: 10.1111/ijd.13322

Chapter 3

Psoriasis and Skin Comorbidities

Florentina Silvia Delli and Elena Sotiriou

Abstract

Psoriasis is a heterogeneous skin disease with many clinical presentations in patients with different medical backgrounds. Medical specialties such as rheumatology, pathology, and cardiology focus lately on the systemic inflammation nature of the psoriatic disease. From the Dermatologist's point of view, the revolution of therapeutic spectrum in many autoimmune skin diseases, as well as the progression noted in physiopathological mechanism, the skin comorbidities became an important issue regarding therapeutic choice.

Keywords: psoriasis, vitiligo, alopecia areata, autoimmune bullous skin diseases

1. Introduction

Psoriasis is not a merely skin disease but rather a multisystemic inflammatory disorder. As such, comorbidities, including but not limited to cardiovascular diseases and metabolic syndrome, play a significant role in therapeutic decision-making. Even though skin comorbidities in patients with psoriasis are common, they are usually neglected. The epidemiology studies and therapy-related literature dominate the recently published relevant data. The pathogenesis of comorbid diseases, either systemic or dermatologic, in patients with psoriasis remains unknown; however, shared inflammatory pathways, cellular mediators, genetic susceptibility, and common risk factors are hypothesized to be contributing elements.

Patients with psoriasis are more likely to have at least one other autoimmune disease [1], including vitiligo [2], alopecia areata [1], and autoimmune bullous diseases [3].

The clinical implications of the most frequent comorbid skin diseases associated with psoriasis are discussed in this chapter.

2. Psoriasis and skin comorbidities

2.1 Psoriasis and vitiligo

Vitiligo is the most common disorder of pigmentation. Although the association of psoriasis and vitiligo has been described since 1890, the interrelationship between the two dermatoses remains debatable. Most of the studies found that 6% of patients with vitiligo develop psoriasis [4, 5] and 2% of patients with psoriasis suffer from vitiligo [4]. Furthermore, a clinical and even dermoscopic challenge is to distinguish vitiligo from the occurrence of hypopigmentation in areas of previously affected psoriatic skin [6]. Healing of psoriatic lesions often leaves hypopigmentation that could simulate vitiligo. There have been cases reported in the literature of psoriatic plaques and guttate lesions strictly localized to the vitiliginous patches (**Figure 1**), and the two dermatoses occurring together without strict colocalization of lesions. In many cases, it is difficult to say which disease starts first, vitiligo, or psoriasis, or may occur at the same time. A retrospective study found that almost 47% of patients having both diseases had separated lesions [7], while, in another study, 34% of patients' psoriatic plaques covered the vitiligo patches [8].

Many hypotheses tried to explain the pathogenesis of vitiligo. These hypotheses consider the role of neural implication, microvascular anomalies, melanocyte degeneration from oxidative stress, defects in melanocyte adhesion, autoimmunity, somatic mosaicism, and genetic influences [9]. Genetic and immunological factors are present in both diseases, psoriasis and vitiligo. A study in China found that both skin diseases share a common genetic locus in the major histocompatibility complex (MHC) [10]. Precisely, the rs. 9468925 in HLA-C/HLA-B is associated with both psoriasis and vitiligo, providing the first substantial evidence that two different skin diseases share a common genetic locus in the MHC. In the molecular etiopathogenesis mechanism of both diseases, Th1 cytokines play a key role. Vitiligo and psoriasis are both chronic inflammatory Th1 type autoimmune diseases with increased TNF-α and interferon γ levels [8]. Otherwise, both share the activation of the Th17 pathway [11]. Even more,

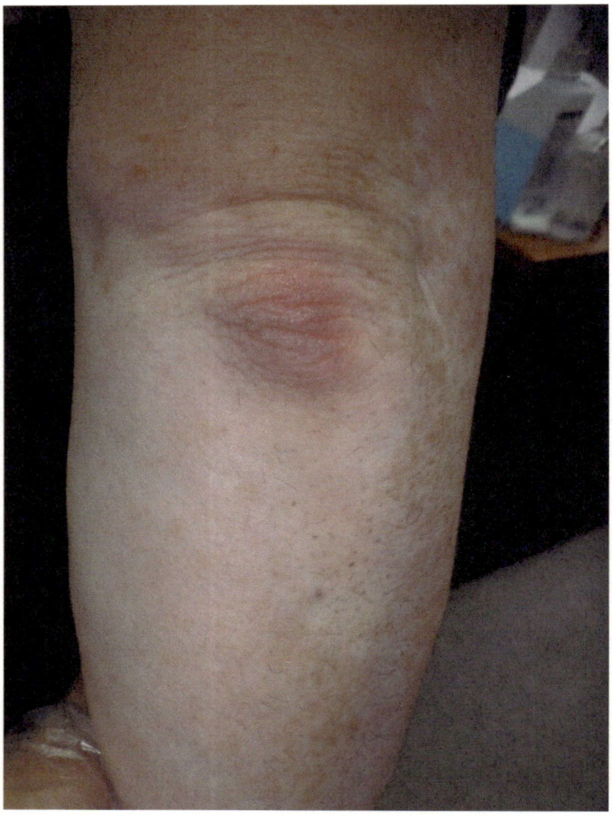

Figure 1.
A typical elbow psoriatic plaque on vitiligo area. Photo from personal collection.

the memory cells might be a link between psoriasis and vitiligo. Recent translational research shows the presence in psoriatic skin of memory CD8+ T cells directed against the melanocyte-derived protein ADAMTSL5 [12], a protein that may favor the development of vitiligo in a predisposed patient. The tissue-resident memory T (T_{RM}) cells are also vital in the recurrence of chronic inflammatory skin disorders, including psoriasis and vitiligo, under pathological or uncontrolled conditions [13].

An interesting phenomenon is the case of vitiligo induced by biological drugs used for psoriasis treatment. The anti-TNF-α (etanercept, infliximab) is one of the most cited groups of biological drugs that induce new-onset vitiligo or progression of pre-existence vitiligo in psoriatic patients [14]. Even anti-IL12/23 [15] and anti-IL17 [15, 16] class can induce a progression of pre-existing vitiligo, while, to date, no cases are reported in the literature considering anti-IL23 drugs. It is difficult to understand how molecules that block cytokines involved in both diseases' pathogenesis can trigger the mechanisms underlying this phenomenon. However, a new type of medication that functions by inhibiting the activity of one or more of the Janus kinase family of enzymes (JAK1, JAK2, JAK3, TYK2), thereby interfering with the JAK-STAT signaling pathway, have been approved for psoriatic therapy and are also a promising novel therapy for vitiligo.

In conclusion, the paucity of data on the link between psoriasis and vitiligo underlines the gaps of knowledge on this topic. To highlight the pathogenetic mechanisms underlying the two diseases are strongly needed further studies.

2.2 Psoriasis and alopecia areata

Psoriatic lesions of the scalp are sometimes associated with symptomatic hair loss and alopecia. The type of alopecia can be, in most cases, characterized using the dermatoscope.

Alopecia areata (AA) is the most common immune-mediated hair loss disorder with a lifetime prevalence of 2% [17]. Early studies of the last decade showed that patients with psoriasis and psoriatic arthritis have a higher risk to develop other autoimmune disorders, particularly alopecia areata (AA) [1, 18]. Two large population studies demonstrated an odds ratio of 2.4 [1, 18].

The Renbeok phenomen, the opposite of the Koebner phenomenon, was originally described in AA patients where hair growth was observed in psoriatic plaques. Generalizing, it is an interesting phenomenon where one skin condition inhibits other skin conditions and confirms once again the complex immunological overlap between these two skin diseases.

In the case of a patient with psoriasis and AA, the complexity of the common immunological paths that share these both skin disorders must be considered when selecting therapeutic regimens, to avoid worsening one of their inflammatory conditions while treating the other. For example, contrary to the initial hope that tumor necrosis factor α (TNFα) may have a role in the pathogenesis of AA, many reports have demonstrated the inefficiency of anti-TNFα drugs in the treatment of AA [19].

Moreover, careful selection of biological treatment regimens may offer therapeutic benefits for both their psoriasis and AA while giving us experience with the newer biologics in AA. The investigation of cytokine profile and the relation between different categories of cytokines is continuing in both psoriasis and AA. A recent example comes from a recent study where the authors conclude that psoriasis T helper type 17 (Th17) cytokines can inhibit some inflammatory processes involved in AA pathogenesis [20].

2.3 Psoriasis and bullous diseases

Autoimmune bullous diseases (AIBD) and more frequent pemphigoid group, often develop in patients with psoriasis. The rare nature of AIBD makes collecting epidemiologic data with a representative number of patients a laborious process. Among the pemphigoid diseases, bullous pemphigoid (BP), the most prevalent subcutaneous autoimmune bullous disease worldwide, is also the most prevalent blistering disease associated with psoriasis. This association has been studied and confirmed on large populations [21–24]. BP and psoriasis do not share any common HLA or otherwise genetic susceptibility. A consequence of epigenetic events related to the psoriatic inflammatory cascade and changes at the basal membrane zone in psoriasis is possible pathogenetic hypotheses, along with increased of certain Th1/Th17 cytokines and chemokines levels that may be another link for their association [25].

Antilaminin γ1 pemphigoid is the second most prevalent AIBD associated with psoriasis, followed by the combination of BP with antilaminin γ1 pemphigoid [26]. The explanation of the subepidermal blister formation in psoriatic patients is mainly provided by Mondello and Vaccaro studies [27, 28]. The cleavage and disruption of laminin 1 and laminin α1 within basal membrane zone, either in apparent normal skin or psoriatic lesion [27, 28], might be the main trigger factor for several antibodies production, such as anti-laminin γ1 and anti bullous pemphigoid antigen 180 (BP180). As a result, the development of BP rash is sometimes observed in psoriatic patients. In the same case series of Ohata et al. [26], three patients presented linear IgA bullous dermatosis and two epidermolysis bullosa acquisita.

The relation between psoriasis and BP seems to be bidirectional. The only published study that confirms that psoriasis occurs significantly more frequently in patients with BP than in the control group, comes from Taiwan [21]. Large population studies in each country are necessary to support this association.

Mucous membrane pemphigoid is also a rare chronic autoimmune disorder characterized by subepidermal blistering that has been observed in patients with psoriasis [29]. The laminin degradation stimulated by matrix metalloprotease 9 released from neutrophil infiltrate in the patients with psoriasis may contribute to decreasing the threshold of autoantibodies against laminin γ1 production [30, 31].

A recent systematic review and meta-analysis evaluating the association between pemphigus and psoriasis confirm this association [32]. However, it is difficult to find common pathways between pemphigus and psoriasis pathophysiologic mechanisms.

3. When psoriasis coexists with other skin diseases

Often chronic skin inflammatory diseases coexist with psoriasis suggesting common pathogenic pathways.

Among them, hidradenitis suppurativa (HS) also exhibits a systemic inflammatory nature with systemic comorbidities similar to psoriasis. The systemic inflammation might explain the observation of a recent study, where it was found that in patients with both HS and psoriasis, the disease diagnosed first tended to take a more severe course than the later diagnosed (**Figure 2**) [33].

Pityriasis rubra pilaris (PRP) is an inflammatory dermatologic disorder of unknown cause, which often is misdiagnosed as psoriasis. However, differentiating between erythrodermic PRP and pustular psoriasis is challenging even histologically. The same treatment is indicated in both diseases, despite the absence of standard

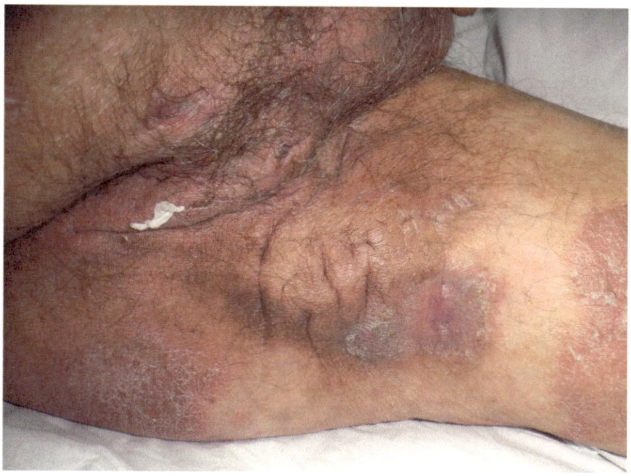

Figure 2.
A 65-year-old male patient. Hidradenitis suppurativa Hurley III coexists with psoriatic plaques. Photo from personal collection.

recommended treatment algorithms for PRP. According to recently published data, we must consider the coexistence of psoriasis and autoimmune diseases in patients with PRP [34]. From our personal experience, a patient can present with erythrodermic PRP and the improvement of the rash might be followed by the appearance of classical plaque psoriasis after treatment with an anti-TNF-α biological agent.

One of the most paradoxical relationships is between psoriasis and atopic dermatitis (AD). The Th17 immune response is dominant in psoriasis and causes neutrophil migration, induction of innate immunity, and increased epithelial metabolism, while Th2 immunity that characterizes AD is dominated by IL-4 and IL-13 cytokines leading to an impaired epidermal barrier, dampened innate immunity, and eosinophil migration. However, the association of AD with psoriasis is not so rare. Both diseases share many characteristics: high prevalence, chronicity, primary skin inflammation, associated comorbidities, important impact on the quality of patient's life due to itch and stigmatization. Some authors consider that the co-occurrence is an overlapping syndrome [35] and others found bidirectional association [36]. In Bozek's study [35] the patients with concomitant AD and psoriasis were frequently boys and overweight and had skin lesions equally distributed throughout the body. Despite the fact that the pathogenesis of psoriasis and AD is different, a family history of atopic disease is a more frequent finding in children with concomitant AD and psoriasis and in children with AD than in children with only AD or psoriasis [35]. Genetics and epigenetics studies with a focus on this topic might provide useful data regarding the particular management of patients with AD and psoriasis.

4. Conclusion

A new research field in many autoimmune skin diseases and the new therapeutic target molecule consequently developed constitutes the base for the addition of autoimmune skin comorbidities on the general list of psoriasis-associated diseases. Evidence increasingly suggests a relation between psoriasis and vitiligo, alopecia areata, and autoimmune subepidermal bullous diseases.

Recognizing all the comorbid disease burden of psoriasis is essential for ensuring comprehensive care of patients with psoriasis.

Conflict of interest

The authors declare no conflict of interest.

Author details

Florentina Silvia Delli* and Elena Sotiriou
First Dermatology Department, Aristotle University of Medical School Thessaloniki, Greece

*Address all correspondence to: delliflorentina@ymail.com

References

[1] Wu JJ, Nguyen TU, Poon KY, Herrinton LJ. The association of psoriasis with autoimmune diseases. Journal of the American Academy of Dermatology. 2012;**67**(5):924-930. DOI: 10.1016/j.jaad.2012.04.039. Epub 2012 Jun 2

[2] Arunachalam M, Dragoni F, Colucci R, Berti S, Crocetti E, Galeone M, et al. Non-segmental vitiligo and psoriasis comorbidity—a case-control study in Italian patients. Journal of the European Academy of Dermatology and Venereology. 2014;**28**(4):433-437. DOI: 10.1111/jdv.12117. Epub 2013 Feb 26

[3] Kridin K, Bergman R. Association between bullous pemphigoid and psoriasis: A case-control study. Journal of the American Academy of Dermatology. 2017;**77**(2):370-372. DOI: 10.1016/j.jaad.2017.02.057

[4] Sharquie KE, Salman HA, Yaseen AK. Psoriasis and vitiligo are close relatives. Clinical, Cosmetic and Investigational Dermatology. 2017;**10**:341-345. DOI: 10.2147/CCID.S142819

[5] Canu D, Shourick J, Andreu N, Gey A, Ballanger-Désolneux F, Barailler H, et al. Demographic and clinical characteristics of patients with both psoriasis and vitiligo in a cohort of vitiligo patients: A cross-sectional study. Journal of the European Academy of Dermatology and Venereology. 2021;**35**:e676-e679

[6] Amico S, Barnetche T, Dequidt L, Fauconneau A, Gérard E, Boursault L, et al. Characteristics of postinflammatory hyper- and hypopigmentation in patients with psoriasis: A survey study. Journal of the American Academy of Dermatology. 2020;**83**(4):1188-1191. DOI: 10.1016/j.jaad.2020.02.025. Epub 2020 Feb 14

[7] Sheth VM, Guo Y, Qureshi AA. Comorbidities associated with vitiligo: A ten-year retrospective study. Dermatology. 2013;**227**(4):311-315. DOI: 10.1159/000354607. Epub 2013 Oct 4

[8] Sandhu K, Kaur I, Kumar B. Psoriasis and vitiligo. Journal of the American Academy of Dermatology. 2004;**51**(1):149-150

[9] Katz EL, Harris JE. Translational research in vitiligo. Frontiers in Immunology. 2021;**12**:624517. DOI: 10.3389/fimmu.2021.624517

[10] Zhu KJ, Lv YM, Yin XY, et al. Psoriasis regression analysis of MHC loci identifies shared genetic variants with vitiligo. PLoS One. 2011;**6**(11):e23089

[11] Yen H, Chi CC. Association between psoriasis and vitiligo: A systematic review and meta-analysis. American Journal of Clinical Dermatology. 2019;**20**(1):31-40. DOI: 10.1007/s40257-018-0394-1

[12] Arakawa A, Siewert K, Stöhr J, Besgen P, Kim SM, Rühl G, et al. Melanocyte antigen triggers autoimmunity in human psoriasis. The Journal of Experimental Medicine. 2015;**212**(13):2203-2212. DOI: 10.1084/jem.20151093. Epub 2015 Nov 30

[13] Chen L, Shen Z. Tissue-resident memory T cells and their biological characteristics in the recurrence of inflammatory skin disorders. Cellular & Molecular Immunology. 2020;**17**(1):64-75. DOI: 10.1038/s41423-019-0291-4. Epub 2019 Oct 8

[14] Anthony N, Bourneau-Martin D, Ghamrawi S, Lagarce L, Babin M,

Briet M. Drug-induced vitiligo: A case/non-case study in Vigibase®, the WHO pharmacovigilance database. Fundamental & Clinical Pharmacology. 2020;**34**(6):736-742. DOI: 10.1111/fcp.12558. Epub 2020 Apr 27

[15] Méry-Bossard L, Bagny K, Chaby G, Khemis A, Maccari F, Marotte H, et al. New-onset vitiligo and progression of pre-existing vitiligo during treatment with biological agents in chronic inflammatory diseases. Journal of the European Academy of Dermatology and Venereology. 2017;**31**(1):181-186. DOI: 10.1111/jdv.13759. Epub 2016 Jun 13

[16] Marasca C, Fornaro L, Martora F, Picone V, Fabbrocini G, Megna M. Onset of vitiligo in a psoriasis patient on ixekizumab. Dermatologic Therapy. 2021;**34**(5):e15102. DOI: 10.1111/dth.15102. Epub 2021 Sep 2

[17] Gilhar A, Etzioni A, Paus R. Alopecia areata. The New England Journal of Medicine. 2012;**366**(16):1515-1525. DOI: 10.1056/NEJMra1103442

[18] Sy C, Chen YJ, Tsteng WC, Lin MW, Chen TJ, Hwang CY, et al. Comorbidities profiles among patients with alopecia areata: The importance of onset age, a nationwide population-based study. JAAD. 2011;**65**(5):949-956. DOI: 10.1016/j.jaad.2010.08.032. Epub 2011 May 25

[19] Strober BE, Siu K, Alexis AF, Kim G, Washenik K, Sinha A, et al. Etanercept does not effectively treat moderate to severe alopecia areata: An open-label study. Journal of the American Academy of Dermatology. 2005;**52**(6):1082-1084. DOI: 10.1016/j.jaad.2005.03.039

[20] Guttman-Yassky E, Nia JK, Hashim PW, Mansouri Y, Alia E, Taliercio M, et al. Efficacy and safety of secukinumab treatment in adults with extensive alopecia areata. Archives of Dermatological Research. 2018;**310**(8):607-614. DOI: 10.1007/s00403-018-1853-5. Epub 2018 Aug 18

[21] Chen YJ, Wu CY, Lin MW, Chen TJ, Liao KK, Chen YC, et al. Comorbidity profiles among patients with bullous pemphigoid: A nationwide population-based study. The British Journal of Dermatology. 2011;**165**(3):593-599. DOI: 10.1111/j.1365-2133.2011.10386.x. Epub 2011 Jul 28

[22] Tsai TF, Wang TS, Hung ST, Tsai PI, Schenkel B, Zhang M, et al. Epidemiology and comorbidities of psoriasis patients in a national database in Taiwan. Journal of Dermatological Science. 2011;**63**(1):40-46. DOI: 10.1016/j.jdermsci.2011.03.002. Epub 2011 Mar 16

[23] Phan K, Goyal S, Murrell DF. Association between bullous pemphigoid and psoriasis: Systematic review and meta-analysis of case-control studies. The Australasian Journal of Dermatology. 2019;**60**(1):23-28. DOI: 10.1111/ajd.12899. Epub 2018 Aug 23

[24] Kridin K, Ludwig RJ, Schonmann Y, Damiani G, Cohen AD. The bidirectional association between bullous pemphigoid and psoriasis: A population-based cohort study. Frontiers in Medicine (Lausanne). 2020;7:511. DOI: 10.3389/fmed.2020.00511

[25] Dainichi T, Kabashima K. Interaction of psoriasis and bullous diseases. Frontiers in Medicine (Lausanne). 2018;5:222. DOI: 10.3389/fmed.2018.00222

[26] Ohata C, Ishii N, Koga H, Fukuda S, Tateishi C, Tsuruta D, et al. Coexistence of autoimmune bullous diseases (AIBDs) and psoriasis: A series of 145 cases. Journal of the American Academy of Dermatology. 2015;**73**(1):50-55

[27] Mondello MR, Magaudda L, Pergolizzi S, Santoro A, Vaccaro M, Califano L, et al. Behavior of laminin 1 and type IV collagen in uninvolved psoriatic skin. Immunohistochemical study using confocal laser scanning microscopy. Archives of Dermatological Research. 1996;**288**(9):527-531. DOI: 10.1007/BF02505249

[28] Vaccaro M, Magaudda L, Cutroneo G, Trimarchi F, Barbuzza O, Guarneri F, et al. Changes in the distribution of laminin alpha1 chain in psoriatic skin: Immunohistochemical study using confocal laser scanning microscopy. The British Journal of Dermatology. 2002;**146**(3):392-398. DOI: 10.1046/j.1365-2133.2002.04637.x

[29] Lee J, Seiffert-Sinha K, Attwood K, Sinha AA. A retrospective study of patient-reported data of bullous pemphigoid and mucous membrane pemphigoid from a US-based registry. Frontiers in Immunology. 2019;**10**:2219. DOI: 10.3389/fimmu.2019.02219

[30] Mezentsev A, Nikolaev A, Bruskin S. Matrix metalloproteinases and their role in psoriasis. Gene. 2014;**540**(1):1-10. DOI: 10.1016/j.gene.2014.01.068. Epub 2014 Feb 8

[31] Dainichi T, Kurono S, Ohyama B, Ishii N, Sanzen N, Hayashi M, et al. Anti-laminin gamma-1 pemphigoid. Proceedings of the National Academy of Sciences of the United States of America. 2009;**106**(8):2800-2805. DOI: 10.1073/pnas.0809230106. Epub 2009 Feb 5

[32] Phan K, Ramachandran V, Smith SD. Association between pemphigus and psoriasis: A systematic review and meta-analysis. Dermatology Online Journal. 2020;**26**(8):13030/qt5g78q4f4

[33] Pinter A, Sarlak M, Zeiner KN, et al. Coprevalence of hidradenitis suppurativa and psoriasis: Detailed demographic, disease severity and comorbidity pattern. Dermatology. 2021;**237**(5):759-768. DOI: 10.1159/000511868

[34] García-Briz MI, García-Ruiz R, Zayas-Gávila AI, et al. Pityriasis rubra pilaris. Something more than a disorder of queratinization? Medicina Cutánea Ibero-Latino-Americana. 2018;**46**(1):7-12

[35] Bozek A, Zajac M, Krupka M. Atopic dermatitis and psoriasis as overlapping syndromes. Mediators of Inflammation. 2020;**2020**:7527859. DOI: 10.1155/2020/7527859

[36] Dai YX, Tai YH, Chang YT, Chen TJ, Chen MH. Bidirectional association between psoriasis and atopic dermatitis: A nationwide population-based cohort study. Dermatology. 2021;**237**(4):521-527. DOI: 10.1159/000514581. Epub 2021 Mar 18

Section 2

Immune System and Psoriasis

Chapter 4

Th17/IL-17, Immunometabolism and Psoriatic Disease: A Pathological Trifecta

Seema Chhabra, Smrity Sahu, Keshav Sharma, Maryada Sharma, Lekha Rani, Ranjana Minz and Sunil Dogra

Abstract

The burgeoning arena of immunometabolism provides evidence of how cellular, as well as local (tissue)/systemic metabolic pathways, are playing an important role in controlling immunity and inflammation. An intricate and elaborate network of various metabolic circuits specifically glycolysis, fatty acid oxidation and synthesis and amino acid metabolism precisely generate metabolites that rewire the immune response. Psoriasis is a chronic progressive self-perpetuated "IL-17-centric" inflammatory disease characterized by the co-existence of autoimmune and autoinflammatory pathways. Metabolic responses, governed by oxygen levels, nutrient availability, growth factors, cytokines, AMP/ATP ratios and amino acids, play a pivotal role in programming Th17 cell fate determination. Understanding the intricate interactions and complex interplay of molecular mechanisms responsible for Th17 cell metabolic rewiring, an important determinant of Th17 cell plasticity and heterogeneity, holds the potential to reshape psoriatic therapeutics in ways currently unimagined. This chapter entails with most recent updates on major cellular and systemic metabolic pathways regulating differentiation of Th17 cells as well their cross-talk with intracellular signaling mediators and also sheds light on how dysregulation of these pathways can be responsible for immune impairment and development of psoriatic disease. A better understanding of these metabolic processes could unveil an intriguing leverage point for therapeutic interventions to modulate metabolic programming and Th17 cell responses in this multi-systemic inflammatory disease.

Keywords: IL-17, Th17 cells, immune-metabolism, psoriasis, psoriatic disease

1. Introduction

Environment-driven metabolic adaptations perform important roles in regulating the immune system. Specific metabolic pathways control T-cell activation/proliferation/differentiation and regulate the switch towards either pro- or anti-inflammatory responses: it, therefore, seems rational that metabolic trepidations can alter self-immune tolerance [1]. Aberrant metabolic pathways constitute a molecular snapshot of the cellular processes that are exaggerated during disease pathogenesis [2]. This immune-metabolic interactome can orchestrate the choreography of interleukin (IL)-17-producing T helper (Th17) cells-induced pathogenicity in psoriatic patients, manifested as a 'psoriatic march', ultimately resulting in the development of a variety of psoriasis-associated co-morbidities [3]. Metabolic anomalies influencing the T regulatory cells (Treg)/Th17 axis play a paramount role in the pathophysiology of psoriasis, so it is imperative to understand the close linkage between metabolic pathways and immune cell function: this may unveil specific interventional targets and suggest indirect dietary styles and repositioning of metabolic drugs that beneficially impact the abnormal T-cell metabolism [4].

2. Th17 cells

Faced with any antigenic stimulus, either an intracellular or extracellular pathogen or any tissue homeostatic alteration, naïve CD4^{+} T-cells respond via activation, proliferation, and finally differentiation into specialized T-effector cell subsets which are specifically programmed to deal with the offending agent/s. One such specialized T-effector cell subset is comprised of Th17 cells, best known as a host-defensive effector T-cell subset at barrier mucosal tissues (intestine, lung, skin) with a prime role in providing immunity against fungi and other extracellular pathogens and in sustaining gut barrier integrity by transdifferentiating into Th1-like or Treg-like cells [5]. Retinoic acid-related orphan receptor-gamma (RORγt), a signature ligand-dependent transcription factor for Th17 cells has been characterized as the molecular orchestrator of Th17 cell program. RORγt belongs to a subfamily of nuclear receptors, encoded by the master switch gene *RORA-C* (or *NR1F1-3*) [6]. A variety of transcriptional regulators of RORγt, as well as other transcription factors that either interact with RORγt or bind the promoter or the intergenic regions of the *IL-17* gene locus, play a crucial role in the generation of Th17 cells (**Figure 1**) [7].

Th17 cells exhibit much superior plasticity compared to other T-cell subsets and epitomize a highly functionally diverse effector T cell population and also display stem cell-associated features [8]. Transforming growth factor (TGF)-β1 and IL-6 induced non-pathogenic/anti-inflammatory Th17 cells have been shown to play an important role in supporting cellular and organismal metabolic homeostasis as well [9]. However, Th17 cells are also recognized for their pathogenicity against the host, due to their association with several autoimmune diseases including psoriasis, multiple sclerosis, rheumatoid arthritis, inflammatory bowel disease, and diabetes mellitus. TGF-β3-induced, IL-23- dependent, functionally distinct pathogenic Th17 cells are characterized by different molecular, biochemical, and metabolic profiles (**Table 1**), conferring a proinflammatory phenotype to this effector T-cell subset [10].

Th17 cell evolution towards pro-inflammatory *vs*. anti-inflammatory or homeostatic phenotype is determined not only by a set of specific polarizing cytokines (TGF-β3 + IL-23 or IL-1β + IL-6 + IL-23 *vs.* TGF-β1 + IL-6) but also by a dynamically changing metabolic milieu comprised by a variety of metabolites *viz*. fatty acids, phospholipids, cholesterol intermediates, oxysterols and amino acids [11–16]. These metabolites drive Th17 plasticity by changing the latter's epigenetic landscape by serving as substrates for chromatin-modifying enzymes [17]. This remarkable metabolic heterogeneity can hugely influenceTh17 cell lineage plasticity and their effector function, thereby impacting the course of Th17-associated autoimmune inflammatory diseases, including psoriasis [18].

DOI: http://dx.doi.org/10.5772/intechopen.102633

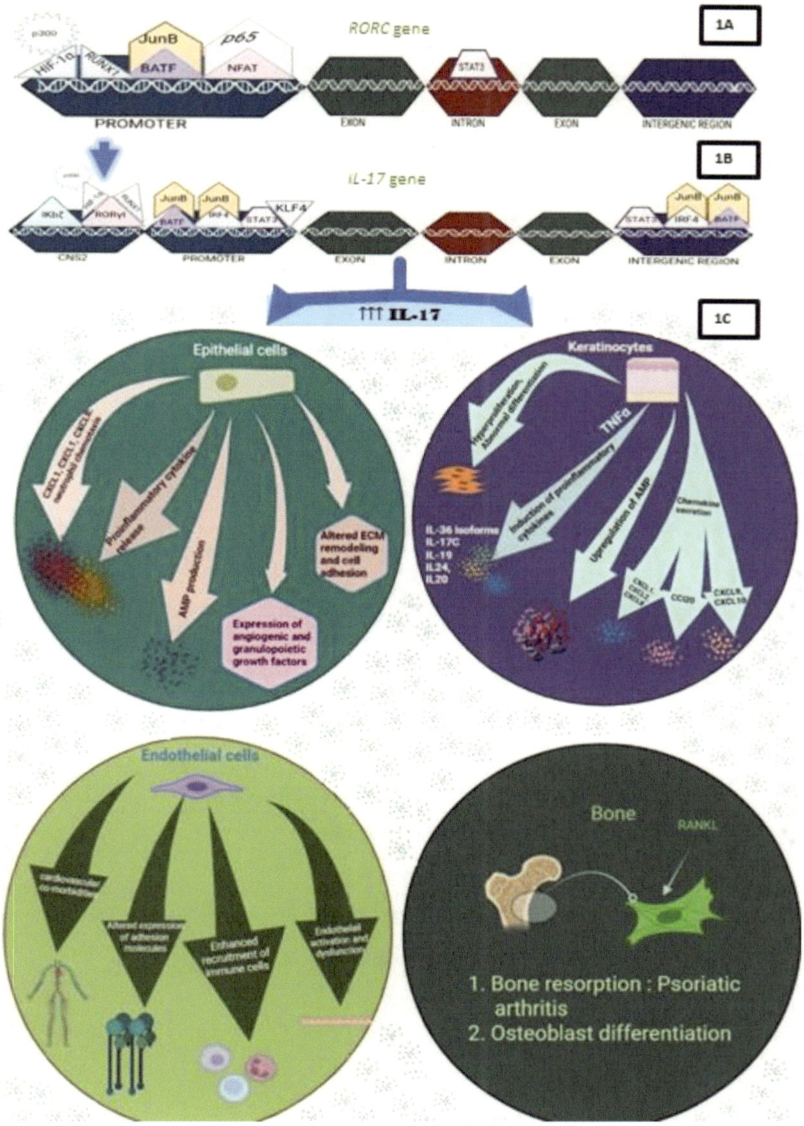

Figure 1.
IL-17 induced "Psoriasogenicity": psoriatic march. (A) A constellation of regulatory factors including hypoxia-inducible factor (HIF)-1α (with recruited factor p300 having histone acetyltransferase activity), runt-related transcription factor (RUNX1), basic leucine zipper ATF-like transcription factor (BATF)- Jun B heterodimer, nuclear factor of activated T cells (NFAT), p65 NF-kB subunit, and signal transducer and activator of transcription (STAT) 3 act as co-operators of RORC gene, enhancing its expression and resulting in increased Th17- lineage-specific transcription factor RORγt. (B) RORγt binds to ROR response elements (RORE) located in CNS2 (conserved non-coding sequences) of the IL-17 gene, and globally controls its transcription. The effect of transcriptional regulator RUNX1 (binding to CNS2 region of IL-17) is also dependent on RORγt; HIF-1α (coactivator for RORγt) physically associates with RORγt promoting IL-17 expression without direct binding on IL-17 locus. Nuclear protein inhibitor of kB (IκB)ζ, is another regulator, that also binds CNS2 elements in the IL-17 locus. Various other transcription regulators that promote IL-17 gene expression by binding to its promoter include BATF, JunB, interferon regulatory factor (IRF)4, STAT3, Kruppel-like factor (KLF) 4. (C) IL-17 leads to induction of various genes encoding for inflammatory mediators, chemokines, antimicrobial peptides, and the osteoclastogenic factor RANKL. This leads to the wide-spread biological effects of IL-17, affecting a variety of cell types/tissues including keratinocytes, endothelial cells, fibroblasts, epithelial cells, and bone.

Parameter	Non-pathogenic Th17 cells	Pathogenic Th17 cells
Polarizing cytokine	TGF-β1/IL-6	TGF-β3 + IL-6 IL-1β + IL-6 + IL-23
Master transcription factor	RORγt	RORγt
Upregulated expression of other relevant genes important for Th17 cell heterogeneity	*IL-10, Ahr, cMaf*	*IL-23, T-bet, CSF2*
CD5L expression	Positive	Negative
Cytokines secreted	IL-17, IL-10, IL-9	IL-17, IFN-γ, GM-CSF
Metabolic profile	Glycolytic ↑	Glycolytic ↑↑↑
	Glutaminolytic ↑	Glutaminolytic ↑↑↑
	Lipogenic (FAS)↑↑↑	Lipogenic (FAS) ↑↑↑
	Cholesterol biosynthesis↑	Cholesterol biosynthesis ↑↑↑
Biochemical profile:		
• Cholesterol & it's derivatives	Low	High
• PUFA levels	High	Low
• SFA/MUFA levels	Low	High
α-KG, 2-HG levels	High ↑	High ↑↑↑
Functional profile	Anti-inflammatory/regulatory	Pro-inflammatory
	Homeostasis/microbiota homeostasis	Autoimmunity
	Tissue repair/barrier integrity	Fibrosis
	Adipogenesis	Tumorigenic
	Thermogenesis	

Ahr, aryl hydrocarbon receptor; c-maf, c-musculoaponeurotic fibrosarcoma expression; csf2, colony stimulating factor; T-bet, T-box expressed in T cells; PUFA, polyunsaturated fatty acids; SFA, saturated fatty acids; MUFA, monounsaturated fatty caids; α-KG, alpha-ketoglutarate; 2-HG, 2-hydroxyglutarate.

Table 1.
Differences between non-pathogenic and pathogenic Th17 cells.

3. Psoriasis/psoriatic disease

Psoriasis is a progressive self-sustained and self-perpetuated inflammatory disease driven by the coexisting autoimmune and autoinflammatory pathways that, while primarily presenting with cutaneous involvement, also manifests as seronegative inflammatory arthritis with synovitis, enthesitis, dactylitis, and spondylitis [19]. It is quite heterogeneous in nature, characterized by a dynamic interplay of the individual's genetic landscape, tissue-specific immune micro-environments, metabolite/immune-metabolite signature, host-microbiome interactions, and biomechanical stressors [20, 21].

3.1 Psoriasis and metabolic syndrome

Psoriasis has long been recognized as a chronic immune-mediated multi-systemic inflammatory disorder, associated with numerous comorbidities *viz.* Crohn's disease, depression, cardiovascular disease, and metabolic syndrome [22]. A concept of 'psoriatic march' was postulated by Boehncke et al. for this inflammatory cascade to highlight the series of systemic inflammatory effects and their relationship with obesity and metabolic syndrome [23]. Metabolic syndrome represents a spectrum of metabolic complications encompassing obesity, hypertension, type 2 diabetes, insulin resistance, atherogenic dyslipidemia and non-alcoholic fatty liver disease (NAFLD) [21]. A recent metanalysis of 63 studies encompassing 15,939 psoriasis patients and 103,984 controls reported a significant association of psoriasis and metabolic syndrome (Odds ratio: 2.077; 95% confidence interval: 1.84–2.34) emphasizing regular monitoring of psoriatic patients for metabolic syndrome complications, including increased fasting plasma glucose levels, raised triglyceride levels, lowered high density cholesterol (HDL) levels, hypertension, and waist circumference [24]. Concurrent occurrence of these metabolic complications in psoriatic patients increases their risk of developing micro and macrovascular adversities contributing to significant morbidity and mortality [25, 26]. Increasing evidence demonstrates a complex interplay among immune cells with attendant aberrant immune dysfunction (such as is seen in psoriasis) and altered cellular and systemic metabolic axes across various organ systems, including adipose tissue, in triggering both local and systemic inflammation [27].

3.2 Th17/IL-17: crucial players in psoriasis

Psoriasis is considered as a "IL-17 centric" disease with a preponderance of pathogenic Th17 cells [28]. Psoriatic Th17 cells produce high levels of IL-17 (A to F), IL-26, IL-29 and IL-22 that synergistically act as transcriptional enhancers of many keratinocyte-expressed genes. IL-26 is linked with increased vascularisation while IL-29 regulates the expression of antiviral proteins [29, 30]. IL-17 induced inflammatory effects are not only limited to cutaneous plaques but also to more distant alterations in numerous different cell types that are responsible for producing systemic inflammatory effects and psoriasis-associated co-morbidities [31]. (**Figure 1**) IL-17 mediated psoriasogenicity is also linked in part to its synergism with other cytokines such as tumor necrosis factor (TNF)-α, IL-22, IL-23, IL-1β, IL-6, TGF-β across various organ systems [32].

4. Immunometabolism

A multifaceted, complex regulation of immune networks both depend on, and influences, cellular and local/systemic metabolic environment. This intricate, dynamic interplay between immunity and metabolism, i.e., "immunometabolism" outlines the metabolic patterning of immune cells and maintains metabolic homeostasis (local/systemic) but can also result in metabolic disorders dominated by deranged immune cells [33, 34]. In other words, immunometabolism can be defined as a molecular and biochemical intertwining of metabolism and immunology in all organisms that accounts for the physiological functioning of the immune system in different metabolic conditions in health and disease [35]. Immune response/inflammation can modulate cellular and tissue/systemic metabolism and vice-versa. Therefore, there are 2 dimensions to immunometabolism: the first is "cellular immunometabolism", which includes the intracellular metabolism of a variety of immune cells under different states of activation, polarization, proliferation, and differentiation and the 2nd dimension is tissue/systemic immunometabolism, which explores the influences of immune cells and their products on local and systemic metabolism across various settings/organs [36]. Thus, the immune system, which can be prompted by the metabolic status of the body can, in turn, have significant consequences on cellular and systemic metabolic homeostasis or disarray.

We will cover these two dimensions of psoriasis-associated immune-metabolism separately:

A. Cellular immunometabolism

The impact of changes in major cellular metabolic pathways on differentiation of Th17 cells, the "signature" cells in psoriasis.

B. Tissue/systemic immunometabolism

The influence of the resultant Th17 response on metabolism across various tissues or organs, especially white adipose tissue (visceral and cutaneous) culminating in metabolic syndrome and other psoriasis-associated co-morbidities.

Before delving deeper into these, we will brush up on immune-metabolic signaling pathways and discuss a basic outline of the major metabolic pathways used by immune cells.

4.1 Metabolic regulation of immune cells

Innate as well as adaptive immune cells have immense malleability to actively respond to different metabolic demands and diverse metabolic microenvironments *via* dynamic regulation of intracellular metabolism in health and disease [37]. Extracellular/environmental cues such as partial pressure of oxygen, oxidative stress, organ-specific pH, nutrient gradients, and disease-dependent fluctuations of the metabolic environment, can shift the metabolic homeostasis of immune cells. Body fluids such as blood and lymph, and the nervous system represent communication conduits for inter-organ coordination; distal communication is executed by the usual messenger molecules (hormones, neurotrophic peptides, cytokines, chemokines, and metabolites) while organelle communication within the cell is carried out by intracellular, spatially organized metabolic processes [38]. These communication networks at various levels orchestrate and harmonize responses to environmental cues/immunological challenges. The signals are sensed by metabolic serine/threonine kinases *viz.* phosphoinositide 3 kinase (PI3K)—protein kinase A, G and C (AGC) kinases (Akt), mechanistic/mammalian target of rapamycin (mTOR) C1/C2, and energy stress pathway kinases, *i.e.,* liver kinase (LK) B1–5′AMP-activated protein kinase (AMPK) in co-ordination with metabolic transcription factors like hypoxia-inducible factor (HIF)-1α, cellular-myelocytomatosis oncogene (c-MYC) and associated nutrient signaling networks. These integrate available environmental information to synchronize cellular proliferation by metabolic revamping [39]. mTOR has been recognized as a molecular orchestrator of immune cell metabolism and catalyzes aerobic glycolysis and anabolic metabolism after stimulation by proinflammatory agents [40]. AMPK, a sensitive radar for decreased cellular nutrients and energy, stimulates catabolic pathways by impeding mTORC1 activity and primarily facilitates T cell adaptation to situations of low nutrient availability as seen during malnutrition, starvation and in hypoxic microenvironments associated with chronic inflammatory conditions [41].

AMPK signaling promotes cell survival and also triggers autophagy (as an energy-preserving mechanism) and mitochondrial biogenesis. HIF-1α, regulated by growth factor signals, oxygen levels, and reactive oxygen species (ROS), rapidly increases in an mTOR-dependent manner and binds to hypoxia response elements (HRE) located in the promoter region of various target genes, this leads to their activation by opening the chromatin structure. Thus, the mTOR/HIF-1α axis is associated with the initiation and development of a "pro-inflammatory" metabolic signature while activation of AMPK favors the generation of an anti-inflammatory/tolerogenic response.

These intertwined and reciprocal PI3K-Akt/mTORC/HIF-1α/c-MYC and LKB1–AMPK immunometabolic signaling networks crosstalk *via* direct reciprocal antagonisms, such as between mTORC1 and AMPK or Akt and LKB1 to regulate metabolism to meet context-specific and cell-specific functional needs [39]. These pathways are also mutually influenced by metabolites and nutrients generated as a consequence of these kinase dependent metabolic signaling, constituting 'bidirectional metabolic signalling' e.g. amino acid availability promoting mTORC1 signaling while low cellular glucose, low glutamine and elevated adenosine monophosphate (AMP) and adenosine diphosphate (ADP) concentrations can activate the AMPK pathway; metabolites generated from mitochondria-associated metabolism, i.e. α- ketoglutarate (α-KG), 2- hydroxyglutarate (2-HG) and acetyl-CoA, can influence transcription of a variety of genes lying in these immunometabolic signaling networks [42].

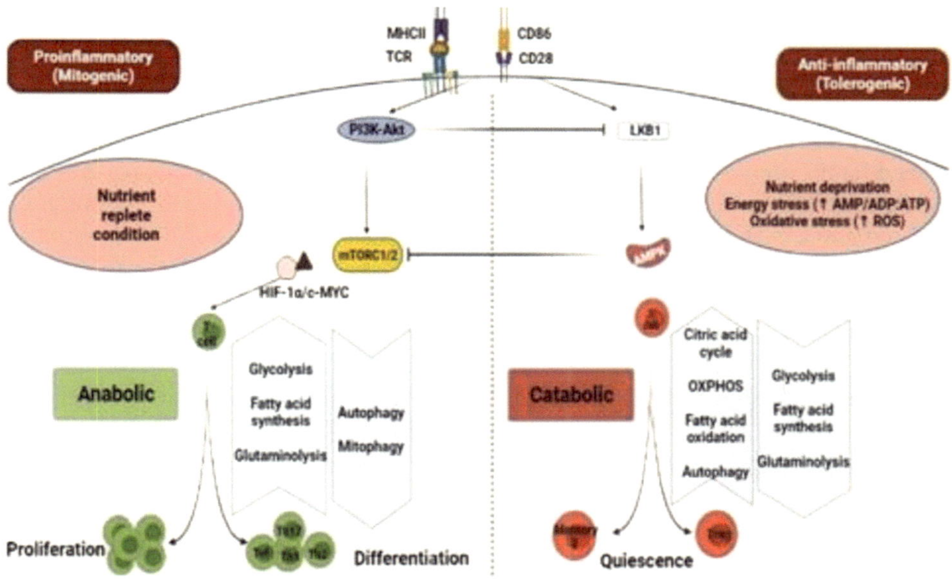

Figure 2.
Signaling pathways regulating immunometabolism of immune cells. T-cell receptor ligation and CD28 costimulatory signals regulate immune-metabolic signaling pathways, i.e., mTORC1/C2 and LKB1-AMPK signaling. These signaling pathways are intertwined and crosstalk via direct reciprocal antagonism, i.e., AMPK directly inhibits mTORC1 while Akt suppresses LKB1 activity. (Left) Nutrient replete conditions activate PI3K-Akt/mTOR signaling that skew metabolic programming towards anabolism-associated processes such as glycolysis, fatty acid synthesis, and glutaminolysis supporting proliferation, differentiation, and heightened immune responses executed by effector immune cells (Th1, Th2, Th17 cells). (Right) Energy stress (increased AMP/ADP:ATP ratio), oxidative stress (increased reactive oxygen species, ROS), nutrient (glucose, glutamine) deprivation during malnutrition/starvation promotes LKB1-AMPK signaling, activating mitochondria-driven oxidative metabolism (citric acid cycle, oxidative phosphorylation, fatty acid oxidation), catabolic programs (autophagy/mitophagy), mitochondrial biogenesis, and inhibiting anabolic programs ultimately resulting in cellular quiescence.

Figure 2 explains how T- cells, under the influence of environmental signals, renew their metabolic equipment to employ metabolic pathways that regulate and propel function of these immune cells.

4.2 Synopsis of metabolic modules used by immune cells

There are 7 fundamental inter-linked and co-regulated metabolic modules employed by immune cells to meet their energy demands. These include glycolysis, pentose phosphate pathway (PPP), citric acid cycle/Krebs cycle, mitochondrial oxidative phosphorylation (OXPHOS)/electron transport chain, fatty acid synthesis (FAS), fatty acid oxidation (FAO), and amino-acid metabolic pathways.

4.2.1 Glycolysis

Once glucose enters the cells through glucose transporters (GLUT), it is rapidly catabolized to pyruvate in a sequential enzymatic process generating a variety of macromolecules needed for different biosynthetic pathways (PPP, *de novo* FAS and amino acid (AA) Hypoxia synthesis pathways) as well as for maintaining cellular redox equilibrium (nicotinamide adenine dinucleotide/nicotinamide adenine dinucleotide hydrogen, NAD+/NADH), thereby supporting anabolic growth. Pyruvate either gets reduced to lactate (*via* lactate dehydrogenase, LDH) by engaging in cytosolic aerobic glycolysis (Warburg effect) in the presence of oxygen, generating 4 molecules of adenosine triphosphate (ATP)/unit of glucose or can enter the mitochondrial matrix (through citrate-pyruvate shuttle system) where it gets oxidized and decarboxylated to acetyl- coenzyme A (CoA) (*via* pyruvate dehydrogenase, PDH) to enter into Kreb's cycle and undergo mitochondrial OXPHOS generating NADH/reduced flavin adenine dinucleotide (FADH2) and a total of 36 molecules of ATP/unit of glucose. Though ATP generation via glycolysis is far less as compared to OXPHOS, activated and effector immune cells rely on glycolysis because of its 100 times faster rate of ATP production, its proficiency to generate a range of biosynthetic intermediates needed for cell growth, as well as its ability to provide both these facilities in oxygen-poor conditions [43]. The mitochondrial enzyme PDH, a key bifurcation enzyme in the choice between glycolytic and mitochondrial oxidative metabolism, in its active dephosphorylated form catalyzes the movement of pyruvate from the cytoplasm to mitochondria for Kreb's cycle. Because of its crucial bifurcating function, PDH is under tight regulation of PDH kinases (PDHKs) that inactivate PDH via phosphorylation, and PDH phosphatases (PDHPs) that dephosphorylate and activate phosphorylated-PDH.

4.2.2 Citric acid cycle/Krebs cycle

Kreb's cycle serves as an important node for multiple nutrient inputs as it integrates fatty acid (FA) and AA metabolism with that of glucose by generating a variety of metabolic biosynthetic intermediates required for FA and AA synthesis and by metabolizing other substrates such as glutamine via glutaminolysis or FAs via β-oxidation. Kreb's cycle results in the generation of different epigenetic-regulating metabolites, e.g., α-KG, 2-HG and acetyl-CoA to calibrate T-cell function [42].

4.2.3 PPP

The PPP provides important precursor molecules for nucleotide synthesis thereby contributing to cell growth. It also generates reducing equivalents of NADPH needed for the maintenance of a favorable cellular redox environment.

4.2.4 Amino acid metabolism

AAs have a significant impact on immune cell metabolism. They contribute to glycolysis by increasing translocation of GLUT1/GLUT4 (by leucine and isoleucine) to the cell surface and also by activating a glycolytic enzyme pyruvate kinase muscle enzyme 2, PKM2 (by serine). Glutaminolysis, i.e., conversion of glutamine into glutamate, is a basic and widespread metabolic process linking OXPHOS, redox regulation, and biosynthetic pathways (protein, nucleotides and branched chain FAs [44]. Glutamate, the first product of glutamine decomposition, can either aid in *de novo* synthesis of glutathione (GSH) to balance oxidative stress, or get converted into α-KG and enter the Kreb's cycle to generate ATP, mitochondrial ROS, and biosynthetic precursors. Hence, the varied end-products of glutamate, by generating counteracting metabolites, i.e., GSH and ROS, enable meticulous synchronization of metabolic flux. AA-derived metabolic products like α-KG and 2-HG assist in chromatin remodeling by affecting histone and DNA modifications [42].

4.2.5 Lipid metabolism

FAs and cholesterol, important building materials for cell membranes, are energy-dense substrates, and are required for post-translational modifications, thereby modulating T-cell proliferation and differentiation. This ability to guide post-translational modifications (by serving as ligands for several transcription factors) varies with the length of their carbon atom chains (short-chain FAs with less than 6 carbon atoms *vs.* long-chain FAs with more than 12 carbon atoms) and their degree of saturation (polyunsaturated fatty acids, PUFA *vs.* saturated fatty acids, SFA/monounsaturated fatty acids, MUFA).

4.2.5.1 Fatty acid synthesis

FAS is chiefly mediated by the enzyme acetyl-CoA carboxylase 1 (ACC1), catalyzing the rate-limiting step in FA biosynthesis, i.e., the carboxylation reaction of acetyl-CoA to malonyl-CoA in the cellular cytoplasm. Acetyl-CoA needed for *de novo* FAS is made available in the cytoplasm through the citrate-pyruvate shuttle that first transfers pyruvate (final glycolytic product) from the cytoplasm into mitochondria to form acetyl-CoA and then transfers a substantial portion of citrate (one of the intermediates generated in the Kreb's cycle by the combination of acetyl-CoA with oxaloacetate) from the mitochondria into the cytosol. In the cytoplasm, citrate lyase generates cytosolic acetyl-CoA from citrate that subsequently powers downstream FA, cholesterol, and lipid biosynthesis [45, 46]. Another important enzyme participating in the initial steps of SFA/MUFA/PUFA generation is fatty acid synthase (FASN), a multienzyme complex that operates downstream of ACC1 and mediates the conversion of acetyl-CoA and malonyl-CoA to saturated long-chain FAs [47].

CD5 antigen-like (CD5L) protein, a member of the scavenger receptor cysteine-rich superfamily inhibits the *de novo* synthesis of SFA through direct binding to FASN, thus helping maintain the intracellular lipidome saturation by modulating PUFA versus SFA levels. CD5L is more than a general inhibitor as it regulates the quantity as well as the quality of fatty acids being generated inside the cell, fine-tuning the FA composition in T cells, causing elevation of PUFA and alterations in specific lipid species, including cholesterol metabolites, guiding post-translational modifications [13].

Acetyl-CoA is a central intermediate in lipid metabolism. In addition to FAS, cytosolic acetyl-CoA can be catalyzed in the mevalonate-cholesterol synthetic pathway, generating cholesterol and its derivatives (desmosterol, 4α-carboxy, 4β-methyl-zymosterol, oxysterols *viz.* 7β, 27-dihydroxy-cholesterol <7β, 27–OHC > and 7α, 27–OHC, 20α-OHC, 22R-OHC, 25-OHC) [15, 48]. All these lipid biosynthetic processes are delicately regulated by coordinated actions of sterol response element binding proteins (SREBPs), the transcription factors which activate all genes necessary for lipid synthesis with SREPB1 inducing genes involved in *de novo* lipogenesis whereas SREBP2 activating genes necessary for cholesterol synthesis and uptake [49].

4.2.5.2 Fatty acid oxidation

Long-chain free FAs enter the metabolizing cells *via* specific transport proteins (SLC27) where they are acted upon by long-chain fatty acid-CoA ligase resulting in a fatty acyl-adenylate, which then reacts with free coenzyme A (CoA) in the presence of acyl-CoA synthetase (ACS) to give an acyl-CoA molecule. Acyl-CoA enters the mitochondria through carnitine transporter, which itself is directed by 3 enzymes including carnitine palmitoyl transferase I (CPT I) located on the cytosolic faces of the outer and inner mitochondrial membranes, and carnitine-acylcarnitine translocase (CAT) and carnitine palmitoyl transferase II (CPT II) located on the interior face of the inner mitochondrial membrane. In the mitochondrial matrix, beta-oxidation cuts the long-chain FAs (now in the form of acyl-CoA molecules) into a series of two-carbon acetate units, which, combined with CoA, form acetyl CoA. This is how acetyl-CoA is added to the cycle, which will be dissipated as carbon dioxide and water, releasing a substantial quantity of energy - captured in the form of ATP—with each beta oxidative cut of the acyl-CoA molecule yielding 5 ATP molecules. It has been calculated that complete β-oxidation of a single palmitate molecule can potentially yield over 100 ATP molecules.

Effector and regulatory/tolerogenic immune cells employ different metabolic modules to fulfill their energy requirements. Activated immune cells and effector immune cell subsets including Th1, Th2, Th17 cells and M1 macrophages upregulate glucose and AA transporters to increase their uptake and rely on aerobic glycolysis, glutaminolysis, PPP and FAS to support pro-inflammatory cytokine secretion while regulatory cells including T regs, memory T cells and M2 macrophages predominantly utilize FAO and OXPHOS to meet their ATP requirements [43].

5. Cellular immunometabolism of Th17 cells, their development and pathogenicity: how intracellular metabolism plays a fundamental role in determining plasticity of Th17 cells

Within Th17 cell subset, depending on the presence of further local stimulatory cues (metabolites), there exists substantial functional and molecular heterogeneity determining the generation of pathogenic or non-pathogenic Th17 cells [18]. Due to the shared developmental requirement of TGF-β and due to functional and physical interaction of master transcriptional factors, i.e. RORγt and Foxp3 regulating Th17 and Treg respectively, these cells are capable of transdifferentiating into each other. The reciprocal metabolic cues are fundamental in shaping the relative proportions of Th17 *vs.* T reg cells and non-pathogenic *vs.* pathogenic Th17 cells, affecting Th17 cell plasticity and pathogenicity. Essentially, the active Th17 cells utilize the faster ATP-producing, oxygen-independent pathways, while the Treg cells utilize the more efficient, if slower, oxidative pathways.

Metabolically, Th17 cells are characterized by *"glycolytic-lipogenic-glutaminolytic"* anabolic phenotype with highly active PPP, ensuring the availability of biosynthetic precursors [50].

5.1 Glycolysis

T cell receptor (TCR) ligation and CD28 co-stimulatory signals induce PI3K dependent phosphorylation of Akt that activates key metabolic regulator mTOR (selective role of mTORC1 but not mTORC2 in Th17 differentiation) leading to increased glycolysis (**Figure 3**). Under Th17-polarizing conditions, the PI3K-Akt/mTORC1/HIF-1α/c-MYC axis activates a series of reactions shifting the Th17/Treg cell balance in favor of Th17 cells. HIF-1α drives Th17 differentiation while simultaneously suppressing Treg induction *via* its differential interaction with transcription factors RORγt and Foxp3 causing transactivation of the former and proteasomal degradation of the latter [51]. HIF-1α doubly enhances this response: firstly, it binds to hypoxia response element (HRE) located in the proximal region of the *RORC* gene promoter (**Figure 1**) and secondly, it might physically associate with RORγt transcription factor, serving as a coactivator for RORγt, thereby increasing *IL-17* gene expression without direct DNA binding on the *IL-17* gene locus [7]. HIF-1α is an essential facilitator of the acquisition of Th17 glycolytic metabolism as shown in **Figure 3** as it enhances expression of a series of glycolytic enzymes including GLUT1 (central glucose transporter on T cells) leading to robust glucose uptake, hexokinase 2 (HK), pyruvate kinase muscle enzyme (PKM2) and lactate dehydrogenase (LDH) causing a shift to aerobic glycolysis. The enzyme PDHK1 that inactivates the PDH enzyme, has been identified as an important player in selective regulation of Th17 cell differentiation and inflammation as evidenced by higher levels of PDHK1 expression on Th17 cells [52]. The transcription factor, inducible cAMP early repressor (ICER, an endogenous repressor of cAMP-responsive element {CRE})-mediated gene transcription, plays a vital role in deciphering Th17 cell biology. It has been shown to be overexpressed in Th17 cells, binds to and suppresses PDHPs, reducing PDH activity thereby enhancing glycolysis, and subsequently increasing Th17 differentiation [53]. Therefore, activation of glycolytic pathways contributes to the differentiation of pro-inflammatory Th17 cells that exhibit enhanced pathogenicity in the context of autoimmune responses.

5.2 Amino acid metabolism

Rapid AA import mediated by the amino acid transporters propels Th17 cell lineage specification by enhancing mTORC1 activity leading to enhanced protein biosynthesis and glycolysis. ICER binds to the *IL-17* gene promoter, enhancing its transcription. It enhances glutaminolysis through glutaminase induction and finally

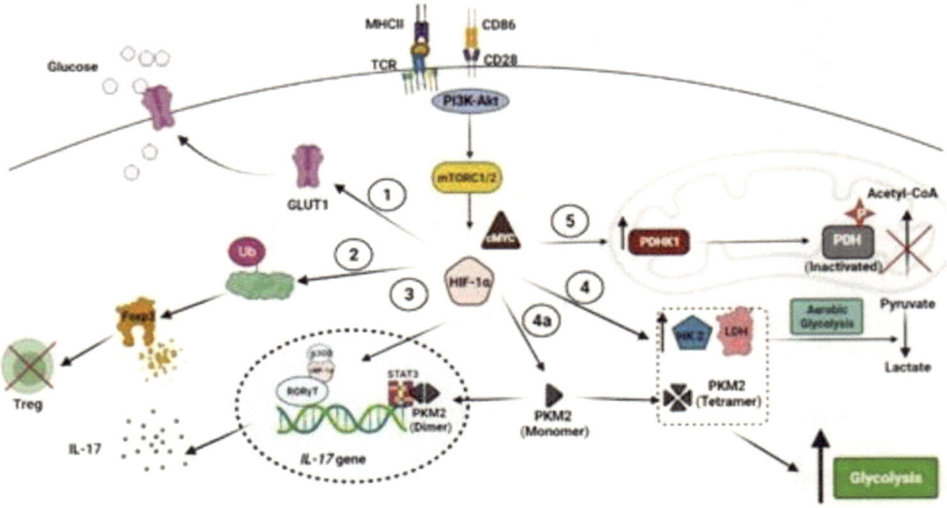

Figure 3.
Impact of glucose metabolism in Th17 cell differentiation: T-cell receptor (TCR) ligation and CD28 co-stimulation integrate phosphatidylinositol 3-kinase (PI3K)-Akt signaling, activating a kaleidoscope of metabolic pathways. mTORC1 activates glycolytic pathways in Th17 cells through activation of the transcription factors c-myc and hypoxia-inducible factor 1-alpha (HIF-1α), mediating multiple pathways. (1) HIF-1α enhances cellular glucose uptake by promoting membrane translocation of the glucose transporter 1 (GLUT1). (2) HIF-1α causes ubiquitination-mediated proteosomal degradation of Foxp3 thereby shifting the Th17/Treg cell balance towards Th17 cells. (3) HIF-1α induces IL-17 gene transcription. (4) HIF-1α enhances expression of genes encoding for key glycolytic enzymes hexokinase (HK2, rate-limiting enzyme of glycolysis), lactate dehydrogenase (LDH, converting pyruvate to lactate), and (4a) pyruvate kinase muscle enzyme 2 (PKM2), that catalyzes the final step of glycolysis producing pyruvate from phosphoenolpyruvate. PKM2 cab functionally exists as either a dimer or a tetramer, each exerting different functions: the cytoplasmic tetrameric configuration is associated with glycolytic activity while nuclear dimeric form interacts with transcription factors and histones, enabling post-translational modifications including the IL-17 gene. (5) HIF-1α also induces pyruvate dehydrogenase kinase, PDHK1 enzyme that phosphorylates and inactivates pyruvate dehydrogenase (PDH) that catalyzes the mitochondrial oxidative conversion of pyruvate to acetyl-coA for launching Kreb's cycle), thereby, nurturing aerobic glycolysis in Th17 cells.

generates glutathione that supports Th17 cell steadiness by enhancing ROS-associated detoxification pathways, polarizing them towards a pathogenic phenotype [54]. Transamination of glutamate (catalyzed by the glutamate oxaloacetate transaminases (GOT)1/2), can epigenetically redirect Th17/T reg equilibrium towards Th17 cell destiny by generating epigenetic-regulating metabolites (α-KG and 2-HG). 2-HG, an inhibitor of α -KG-dependent histone/DNA demethylases, directly increases DNA methylation at CpG islands at the *Foxp3* gene locus leading to its transcriptional repression (**Figure 4**). This is how increased levels of 2-HG in Th17 cells lead to blockade of Treg cell lineage commitment. Th17 cells are characterized by an abundance of α-KG and 2-HG. This highlights the importance of the glutamate-GOT1/2-α-KG-2-HG axis in guiding Th17 cell destiny. GOT1 also contributes to increased mTORC1 signaling by suppressing AMPK activation [55].

Methionine-derived S-adenosyl methionine (SAM) plays a crucial role in chromatin remodeling by serving as a co-factor for epigenome-modifying enzymes, maintaining permissive H3K4me3 marks on *IL-17a*, *IFNG*, and *CSF2* genes promoting their transcription leading to increased pathogenic Th17 generation [56].

In this way, amino acids regulate energy metabolism, redox balance, and impact the epigenetic landscape, modulating Th17 lineage heterogeneity and plasticity [42].

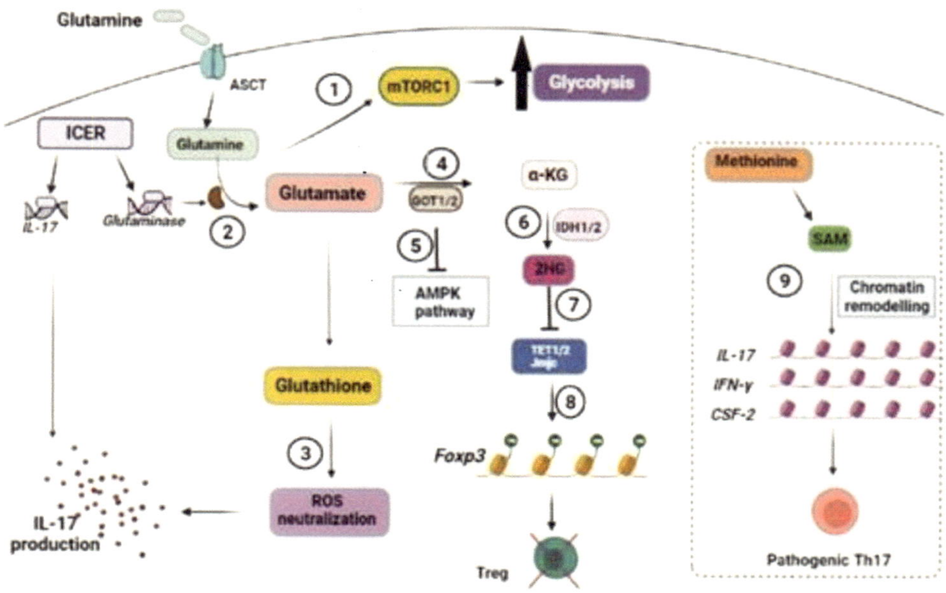

Figure 4.
Glutamine and methionine potentiating Th17 cell differentiation by impacting epigenetic landscape: (1) glutamine imported by the amino acid transporter, (alanine-serine-cysteine transporter, ASCT2) activated mTORC1/c-Myc signaling axis, enhancing glycolysis. (2) Glutaminase, transactivated by ICER binding, generates glutamate and finally glutathione. (3) glutathione causes reactive oxygen species (ROS) neutralization, enhancing pathogenic Th17 cell production. (4) glutamate is metabolized to α-KG [via glutamate oxaloacetate transaminases, GOT1/2]. (5) GOT1/2 inhibits the AMPK pathway leading to enhanced mTORC1 signaling. (6) α-KG generates 2-HG via. Isocitrate dehydrogenases 1/2(IDH1/2). (7) 2-HG impacts DNA methylation by inhibiting histone/DNA demethylases, e.g., Jumonji domain-containing demethylase (Jmjc) and ten-eleven translocation (TET1/2) methylcytosine dioxygenases (that demethylate the CpG islands on the Foxp3 promoter) (8). This leads to heightened DNA methylation at CpG islands of the Foxp3 gene locus and its transcriptional repression. (9) methionine-derived S-adenosyl methionine (SAM), by serving as a methyl donor, causes chromatin remodeling and helps maintain permissive H3K4me3 marks on IL-17, IFNG, and CSF2 genes promoting their transcription, leading to increased pathogenic Th17 generation.

5.3 Lipogenesis

Rather than utilizing already-available exogenous FA for their lipid requirements, Th17 cells primarily engage in the ATP-costly process of *de novo* FAS for their proliferation and differentiation [45]. *De novo* FA and cholesterol synthesis promote activation-induced proliferation and differentiation of Th17 cells (**Figure 5**). Cholesterol precursors, as well as its derivatives, are essential for Th17 cell lineage commitment [57]. They enhance the transcriptional activity of RORγt by increasing co-activator recruitment leading to enhanced *IL-17* and *IL-23* gene transcription (**Figure 5** Inset) CYP51 and CYP27A1, key mediators of the cholesterol biosynthesis pathway are the most highly upregulated genes in Th17 cells [15]. An upregulation of cholesterol biosynthesis and simultaneous downregulation of cholesterol metabolism and efflux during Th17 differentiation leads to the accumulation of the cholesterol precursors desmosterol and its sulphate conjugates. Th17-polarizing milieu upregulates expression of *SREBP1* and *SREBP2*, *FASN*, *3- hydroxy-3-methylglutaryl-CoA reductase (HMGCR*, the rate-limiting enzyme in the mevalonate–cholesterol pathway) as well as expression of enzymes involved in citrate-pyruvate shuttle system leading to enhanced cholesterol synthesis and rapid *de novo* FAS from glucose. This metabolic alteration is again under

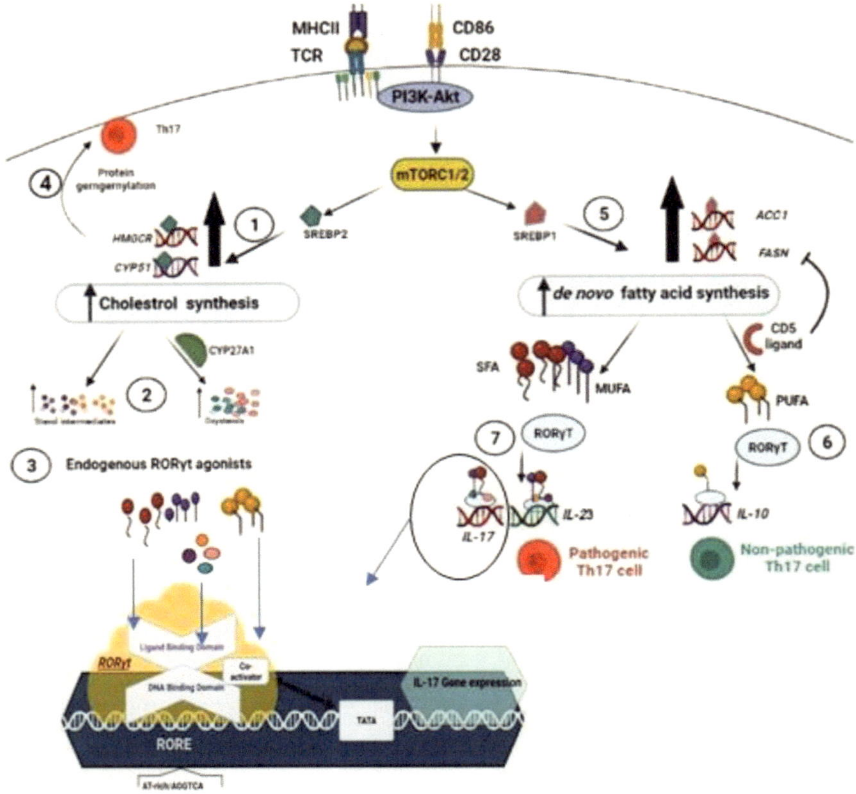

Figure 5.
Lipid metabolism as a central controller of Th17 cell differentiation: T-cell receptor (TCR) ligation and CD28 co-stimulation activate PI3K-Akt/mTORC1 signaling affecting lipid metabolism. (1) increased expression of sterol response element-binding proteins (SREBP2), CYP51 and 3-hydroxy-3-methylglutaryl-CoA reductase (HMGCR) enhances cholesterol biosynthesis. (2) this leads to accumulation of the cholesterol precursors desmosterol, its sulphate conjugates as well as oxysterols [with participation of CYP27A1]. (3) these precursors and derivatives serve as endogenous RORγt agonists, enhancing pathogenic Th17 cell production. The ligand-binding domain (LBD) of RORγt binds to these agonistic ligands including CD5L-dependent displacing the co-repressors and recruiting co-activator proteins, causing enhanced IL-17 gene expression. DNA-binding domain (DBD) of RORγt binds to ROR response elements (RORE) located in CNS2 (conserved non-coding sequences) of IL-17 gene, and globally controls its transcription. (4) HMGCR also contributes towards protein geranylation by generating mevalonate. (5) increased expression of SREBPI stimulates de novo fatty acid synthesis by enhancing the expression of acetyl-CoA carboxylase 1 (ACC1) and fatty acid synthase (FASN) genes. (6) CD5 antigen-like (CD5L) protein inhibits the de novo synthesis of saturated and monounsaturated fatty acids (SFA/MUFA) causing elevation of polyunsaturated fatty acids (PUFA) that results in enhanced RORγt binding to the IL-10 locus leading to its transactivation and production of non-pathogenic Th17 cells. (7) loss of CD5L elevates intracellular SFA/MUFA levels causing enhanced RORγt binding to the IL-17α and IL-23 loci leading to their transactivation and production of pathogenic Th17 cells.

partial control of mTORC1 activation. In addition, to enhancing glycolysis, mTOR signaling fabricates a closely-interacting loop between glycolysis and lipogenesis, "the glycolytic-lipogenic pathway" in Th17 development [58].

5.3.1 Type of fatty acids governing pathogenicity of T cells

Cellular lipid composition influences both generation as well as pathogenicity of Th17 cells. *CD5L* gene, encoding CD5L protein, a "negative" regulator of Th17 pathogenicity; has been recognized as a critical molecular switch of Th17 cell's function (pathogenic versus non-pathogenic phenotype) though it does not affect Th17 differentiation [59]. Loss of CD5L transforms non-pathogenic Th17 cells into disease-inducing pathogenic ones by modulating intracellular lipidome saturation (PUFA versus SFA lipid balance) and by elevating intracellular free cholesterol, thereby regulating the quality and/or quantity of available ligands for RORγt [13]. PUFA regulates the ligand-dependent function of RORγt: in the absence of CD5L/PUFA (**Figure 5**), RORγt binding to the *IL-17* and *IL-23* loci is increased leading to transactivation of both these genes, while binding to *IL-10* locus is decreased leading to its downregulation. Thus, the balance of lipid saturation contributes to CD5L-dependent regulation of Th17 cells by regulating the RORγt genomic binding and Th17-cell transcriptome.

Dietary LCFAs enhance Th1 and Th17 cell differentiation and also alter the composition of the gut microbiome whereas SCFAs (derived from diet/intestine/microbiota) promote Treg cell formation, demonstrating unique phenotypes driven by different fatty acids [60].

The same glycolytic-lipogenic-glutaminolytic metabolic axis co-ordinated by mTORC1/HIF-1α, plays an equally important role in controlling the generation as well as the "pathogenicity" of Th17 cells. These findings highlight how the generation of Tregs/non-pathogenic Th17/pathogenic Th17 cells is tightly linked to their metabolic state, offering potential new targets for the regulation of these two reciprocally regulated T cell subsets (**Table 2**). Thus, it is quite clear that the generation of Th17 cells is entwined with complex and intricate intracellular metabolic adaptations.

Metabolic adjustments favoring Th17 differentiation	Metabolic adjustments impairing Th17 differentiation
Activation of PI3K/AKT-mTORC1 pathway	Activation of AMPK with 5-aminoimidazole-4-carboxamide riboside, AICAR (a direct activator) and metformin
Induction of transcription factors HIF-1α and c-MYC (c-MYC initiates the metabolic reprogramming while HIF-1α sustains it)	Inhibition of glycolysis with 2-deoxyglucose (an inhibitor of all hexokinases)
Activation of glycolysis, pentose-phosphate pathway and glutaminolytic pathway	Inhibition of hexokinase-2 with specific inhibitor 3-bromopyruvate
Selective expression of PDHK1 (inhibited PDH activity) directing pyruvate flow through LDH-mediated reactions to produce lactate (aerobic glycolysis)	Inhibition of acetyl CoA carboxylase 1 with a pharmacological inhibitor soraphen A, inhibiting *de novo* fatty acid synthesis
Overexpression of inducible cAMP early repressor (ICER) that suppresses expression of PDHPs leading to reduced PDH activity and enhanced glycolysis	Inhibition of 3- hydroxy-3-methylglutaryl-CoA reductase (HMGCR) with statins
A diet low in cholesterol and high in fibers can skew Th17 cells towards non-pathogenic anti-inflammatory phenotype	Inhibition of glutamine oxaloacetate transaminase (GOT1/2) by aminooxyacetic acid that leads to decreased production of α-ketoglutarate and 2- hydroxyglutarate skewing Th17 differentiation to the inducible T regulatory cells (iTregs) lineage
A diet high in glucose/salt/ methionine can induce the generation of pathogenic pro-inflammatory Th17 cells	

Table 2.
Comprehensive list of metabolic changes determining Th17 cell fate.

5.4 Crosstalk between IL-17 and cellular immunometabolism in psoriasis

IL-17 has the potential to temper the cellular metabolism in a variety of ways. IL-17 has already been shown to regulate metabolism in psoriatic keratinocytes by reprogramming the urea cycle resulting in excessive polyamine generation that facilitates self-RNA sensing by immune cells independent of RNA-binding proteins LL37 and HNRNPA1 (the proven autoantigens) ultimately leading to amplification of inflammatory circuits [61, 62].

IL-17 also induces intracellular cholesterol accumulation that facilitates NF-κB mediated up-regulation of CCL20, IL-8 and S100A7 expression in keratinocytes thereby further intensifying IL-17A induced psoriatic inflammation [63]. This highlights that how IL-17-induced metabolic alterations can actively participate in eliciting infiltration and activation of innate and adaptive immune cells and keratinocyte hyperproliferation leading to sustained inflammatory dermatoses.

5.4.1 Therapeutics in psoriasis

Depending upon disease severity (based on PASI scores), topical therapy (vitamin analogues, tars, corticosteroids, dithranol, and retinoids), phototherapy (UV-B or PUV-A), and systemic therapy are considered for treatment of psoriasis. Systemic therapeutic agents used in psoriasis include methotrexate, cyclosporine, retinoids and biologics including etanercept, adalimumab, efalizumab, and alefacept. Other approved biologics for psoriasis include anti-IL-23 antibodies (ustekinumab, guselkumab, tildrakizumab, mirikizumab, risankizumab) targeting only IL-23/IL-17 axis and anti-IL-17 antibodies including anti-IL-17A agents (ixekizumab and secukinumab), anti-IL-17 receptor molecules (brodalumab); or drugs targeting both IL-17A and IL-17F (bimekizumab) [64]. These antibodies have shown promising results in the treatment of psoriasis with IL-17 blockers showing much quicker clinical efficacy resulting in a 50% decline in PASI scores as early as 1.8 weeks as compared to IL-23 blockers [65, 66].

To decrease toxicity and enhance efficacy, a few anti-metabolites are currently being repurposed and investigated as potential therapeutic agents for the management of psoriasis [67]. Metformin, an antidiabetic drug, has the potential to exert an antipsoriatic effect via. AMPK activation [68]. Simvastatin, an HMG-CoA reductase inhibitor, in combination with steroids, has demonstrated positive clinical outcomes in psoriatic patients in terms of improved PASI and dermatological life quality index [69]. These examples provide insight to clinicians for investigating the safety and efficacy of existing anti-metabolite drugs to reposition them as effective psoriasis therapeutic agents.

6. Adipose tissue and systemic immunometabolism

One tissue that has recently become an area of intense metabolic research is adipose tissue. The adipose tissue is an important metabolic organ that regulates the balance of energy intake and consumption and is actively involved in the regulation of many systemic metabolic pathways including glucose and lipids. Adipose tissue also serves as an endocrine organ (secreting bioactive adipocytokines) and an important immune cell niche (secreting chemokines and cytokines, exerting beneficial or detrimental effects on immunometabolism) with visceral white adipose tissue as the major immune-metabolic communication hub. Adipose tissue also communicates with other organs including the liver and muscle and contributes to systemic metabolism *via* secretion of a variety of bioactive molecules as mentioned above [70]. Adipose tissue (visceral as well as cutaneous) has recently emerged as an important node linking immunity/inflammation, obesity and a cluster of metabolic diseases including psoriasis. Adipose tissue is a highly dynamic tissue showing the extreme degree of plasticity and remodeling potential (by expansion or contraction of adipocytes in response to energy surplus or famine) that makes it a suitable centre for maintaining immune-metabolic homeostasis [71].

6.1 Adipose tissue and immune-metabolism: an interesting interlink

Besides metabolically active parenchymal adipocytes and preadipocytes, adipose tissue is also comprised of a diverse and malleable immune-landscape comprising both innate and adaptive immunocytes residing in special adipose niches [72]. This diversity of T cell pools in adipose tissue is the result of intracellular metabolic alterations that in turn influence systemic metabolism in innumerable ways. Adipose tissue-resident immune cells include T cells, B cells, macrophages, and dendritic cell subsets and other unconventional lymphocyte subtypes *viz.* invariant natural killer T (iNKT) cells, mucosal-associated invariant T (MAIT) cells, γδ T cells and innate lymphoid cells 2 (ILCs) with either stimulating or regulatory roles under different physiological or pathological conditions [73]. All these immunocytes work in close co-operation with preadipocytes, adipocytes, endothelial cells and stromal cells (fibroblasts) to maintain the immune and metabolic homeostasis of adipose tissue, providing a steady environment to maintain the normal systemic metabolism of an organism [74]. Extremely heterogeneous mesenchymal stromal cells (five subtypes numbered 1–5, defined by single-cell transcriptomics analysis and cytofluorimetric assessment of marker expression) in visceral white adipose tissue have been characterized as key orchestrators of metabolic-immunologic cross-talk by their ability to balance *'immunocyte'* numbers through secretion of IL-33 (subtypes 1–3) and *'adipocyte'* numbers/activities through regulation of adipocyte precursors (subtypes 4 and 5) [75]. The stromal cell-derived IL-33, a mechanosensitive chemokine, dampens aberrant inflammation by increasing Treg numbers. IL-33 has been recently shown to induce mitochondrial rewiring, thereby promoting differentiation of alternatively activated macrophages finally leading to resolution of inflammation [76]. Taken together, tight and well-balanced cooperation and coordination exist between parenchymal-stromal-immune cell populations that ultimately regulate adipose tissue homeostasis.

Intradermal adipocytes residing in "superficial subcutaneous adipose tissue" or "dermal white adipose tissue" of psoriatic skin secrete monocyte chemoattractant protein-1 (MCP-1) favoring macrophage recruitment via the C-C chemokine receptor 2 (CCR2) pathway and also release high levels of antimicrobial peptides, cathelicidin, contributing to the pathophysiology of psoriasis [77].

6.1.1 Adipocytokines and cytokines released by adipocytes

Adipocytes participate in the regulation of the immune system *via* secretion of various cytokines – including IL-6 – and adipocytokines such as adiponectin and leptin. IL-6, an obligatory pro-inflammatory cytokine, drives naïve $CD4^+$ T cells differentiation into Th17 lineage, and in association with IL-17A, regulates the differentiation of adipocytes and their capacity to secrete adipocytokines (especially leptin) and chemokines [78].

Adiponectin is an insulin-sensitizing anti-inflammatory adipocytokine that corrects insulin resistance and obesity-induced NAFLD (21). Leptin is a critical hormonal regulator of metabolism and an important signaling transducer that activates JAK2 kinase causing tyrosine phosphorylation of various downstream signaling proteins, e.g., STAT3, SHP2, IRS2, and PI3K, thereby regulating transcription of genes essential for energy intake and lipid metabolism [79, 80]. Leptin also affects various immune cells including dendritic cells (DCs), neutrophils, NK cells, T and B cells, through surface leptin receptors and regulates a variety of cellular biological processes involving chemokinesis, chemotactic responsiveness, cell migration, proliferation, cell survival (delayed apoptosis) and pro-inflammatory cytokine production [81, 82]. Resistin, another cytokine is also known as an adipose tissue-specific secretory factor (ADSF) also has the pro-inflammatory potential [83].

A disturbed balance of pro-inflammatory and anti-inflammatory cytokines and adipocytokines (hormones) can cause chronic adipose tissue inflammation resulting in obesity and associated metabolic complications.

6.2 Obesity, systemic immunometabolism and psoriasis

Obesity (fat and weight gain/body mass index (BMI) $\geq$ 35 kg/m^2/increased abdominal fat mass) resulting from adipose tissue expansion and adipocyte hypertrophy, is a state of chronic systemic low-grade inflammation that accelerates obesity-related insulin resistance (IR), leading to the development of the metabolic syndrome, including diabetes mellitus (DM). Obesity increases the body's vulnerability to a variety of immune diseases, such as psoriasis, by abnormally altering the whole biology of adipose tissue including stromal-driven regulation of immunocyte and adipocyte numbers. Obesity evokes extensive remodeling of adipose tissue morphology and function with alterations of both immune as well as stromal cell landscapes resulting in metabolic and/or immunologic aberrancies [84]. The number of pro-inflammatory immunocytes *viz.* CD8$^+$ T cells, M1 macrophages, neutrophils, mast cells, and $\gamma\delta$ T cells increases while the proportions of tolerogenic/immunosuppressive cells *viz.* Tregs, regulatory B cells (B regs), eosinophils, iNKT cells, alternatively activated macrophages and type 2 ILCs (copiously producing anti-inflammatory cytokines IL-10, IL-15, IL-2, IL-5, and IL-25) are either decreased or have impaired functional capacity. Various studies have already shown a strong "dose-dependent" relationship between PASI scores and obesity with improvement in disease severity as a result of weight loss in psoriatic patients [85, 86].

Obesity has been postulated to worsen psoriasis *via.* Its effect on the Treg/Th17 axis through various metabolites, adipocytokines like leptin and pro-inflammatory cytokines like IL-6, released by inflamed adipocytes [72, 87, 88] for example, higher leptin and resistin concentrations have been observed in obese, psoriatic patients [89, 90].

Adiponectin plays a crucial role in controlling psoriasiform dermatosis by reducing Th17 cell differentiation, restraining glycolysis in an AMPK dependent fashion, thus tightly regulating their nutritional demands and metabolic function [91–93]. Psoriasis patients with or without metabolic abnormalities exhibit significant hypoadiponectinemia (negatively corelated with psoriasis area severity index, PASI) and hyperleptinemia with leptin resistance (positively corelated with PASI), that contribute to the development of the metabolic syndrome.

The pro-inflammatory cytokine IL-17, a potential linker between metabolic syndrome and psoriasis, causes adipose tissue inflammation by mediating important interactions between adipose tissue and the immune system, leading to IR (the key component of metabolic syndrome) finally manifesting as obesity, DM, hypertension, NAFLD, and hyperlipidemia [21].

Thus, it can be inferred that obesity-driven immune and stromal landscape alterations in adipose tissue, in turn leading to disturbances in systemic metabolism might enhance Th17 differentiation and effector function, consequently leading to increased severity of psoriasis.

6.3 Nutritional metabolism and psoriasis

Beyond the adipose tissue, the diet or nutritional status, a.k.a. nutritional metabolism, also has a profound impact on the immune system by influencing the immune cell metabolic parameters; malnutrition is clearly associated with diminished immune function whereas a "Western" lifestyle/nutritional pattern rich in calories, fat, and salt, leads to a low-grade systemic inflammation thereby predisposing individuals to a variety of autoimmune diseases associated with metabolic complications, including psoriasis. Diet-associated obesity by increasing availability of extracellular lipids revamps cellular metabolism of innate as well as adaptive immune cells [94]. It is quite tantalizing to consider dietary interventions like fasting-mimicking diets and diets low in salt and calories re-stabilizing the immune-metabolism in psoriasis patients, potentially serving as viable substitutes or adjuvants to drugs directly targeting cellular metabolism.

Understanding the relationship between nutrition and metabolism and its impact on cellular/systemic immunometabolism in psoriasis is important to develop novel therapeutic strategies.

7. Metabolomics in psoriasis

Metabolites/biochemical intermediates/end-products, unique chemical fingerprints of proteomic or cellular metabolic pathways, are viewed as keystones of life as they provide vital communication signals that are necessary to sustain life. Metabolomics, a systematic study of the global metabolite profile in a biological system, i.e., cell, tissue, organ, or organism, provides an "instantaneous snapshot"/direct "functional readout of the physiological state", capturing the metabolic perturbations driving physiological and disease states. The metabolome, highly dynamic like transcriptome and proteome, and a rapid indicator of biological status, refer to the complete set of diverse small-molecules (<1500 Da) such as sugars, nucleotides, amino acids and lipids in any biological system.

A large number of psoriatic disease-related metabolomic studies have been carried out in the recent past to identify metabolomic biomarkers associated with psoriatic disease [95]. The majority of studies have focused on identifying a metabolic profile that can be used for diagnosis of psoriasis and/or psoriatic arthritis while others have explored correlating the metabolome with different dimensions of psoriatic disease activity to improve clinical management. A variety of biological samples including peripheral blood (whole blood, plasma, serum, peripheral blood mononuclear cells), urine, and skin tissue (uninvolved skin, psoriatic skin, and corticosteroid treated psoriatic skin) have been researched in these metabolomic studies, revealing alterations predominantly in pathways associated with lipid and amino acid metabolism. To get more meaningful information, a few study-groups have compared metabolite concentrations in different biological milieu by examining metabolomes across multiple sample matrices. A variety of metabolites in the eicosapentaenoic, docosahexaenoic and arachidonic acid pathways are elevated in both the skin and the peripheral blood of psoriatic patients [96, 97]. Plasma and psoriatic skin choline levels correlated positively while citrulline levels across both sample matrices correlated negatively with disease activity scores [98].

A step further, Tarentini et al. integrated results of metabolomic profiling and cytokine/chemokines profiling from lesional skin and serum of psoriatic patients and identified immuno-metabolic clusters indicating biochemical pathways associated with the initial phases of psoriasis development, thus hinting at putative biomarkers of new-onset psoriasis [99].

8. Future perspectives and summary

It is intriguing to explore and validate metabolomic biomarkers that can accurately and reliably predict which psoriatic patients will develop psoriatic arthritis. Identifying metabolites that could differentiate psoriatic arthritis patients from patients with other inflammatory arthritides would be a great added advantage. The synovial fluid, being in direct contact with articular cartilage, bone and synoviocytes, is a very promising candidate for deciphering metabolomic information which can serve as a promising source of biomarkers for psoriatic arthritis.

Metabolic health and gut microbiome dysbiosis are emerging areas of intense investigation as the gut microbiome influences host immunity and metabolism by producing numerous compounds [100]. The connection between the microbiome and the metabolome of patients with heterogenous psoriatic disease holds the potential to highlight aberrant signaling pathways likely driving "psoriatic march". This could pave the path for the development of clinically useful biomarkers for early recognition and management of comorbidities for this patient population [101].

Thus, immuno-metabolic reprogramming may be worth further exploration for the comprehension of its therapeutic potential in psoriasis. In future studies, it will be quite intriguing to define the interplay between IL-17–driven metabolic reprogramming and epigenetics/chromatin remodeling that are responsible for chronic, sustained transcriptional responses seen in psoriasis, which in turn modulate the activity of IL-17- related proinflammatory cytokine programs.

Integrating metabolomics with other high-throughput-omic technologies such as genomics, epigenomics, transcriptomics, and proteomics can unravel molecular, cellular, and functional signatures associated with psoriasis pathogenesis [102, 103]. The "omics" datasets, thus generated, can help construct predictive or diagnostic classifiers, grouping psoriatic patients based on their probability of developing systemic comorbidities or their likelihood to respond to a specific therapy [104]. This cutting-edge, systemic, and holistic approach will allow the clinicians to institute tailored, targeted, precision medicine, based on individual patient characteristics thereby maximizing efficacy and minimizing toxicity and at the same time overcoming the biggest challenge we face in achieving long-term, stable remission in psoriatic patients.

Conflict of interest

None.

Author details

Seema Chhabra[1*], Smrity Sahu[1], Keshav Sharma[1], Maryada Sharma[2], Lekha Rani[1], Ranjana Minz[1] and Sunil Dogra[3]

1 Department of Immunopathology, Postgraduate Institute of Medical Education and Research, Chandigarh, India

2 Department of Otolaryngology and Head and Neck Surgery, Postgraduate Institute of Medical Education and Research, Chandigarh, India

3 Department of Dermatology, Postgraduate Institute of Medical Education and Research, Chandigarh, India

*Address all correspondence to: drseemachhabra@gmail.com; chhabra.seema@pgimer.edu.in

References

[1] Wilson CS, Stocks BT, Hoopes EM, Rhoads JP, McNew KL, Major AS, et al. Metabolic preconditioning in CD4+ T cells restores inducible immune tolerance in lupus-prone mice. JCI Insight. 2021;**6**(19):e143245. Available from: https://pubmed.ncbi.nlm.nih.gov/34403367

[2] Piranavan P, Bhamra M, Perl A. Metabolic targets for treatment of autoimmune diseases. Immunometabolism. 2020;**2**(2):e200012. DOI: 10.20900/immunometab20200012

[3] Wagner A, Wang C, Fessler J, DeTomaso D, Avila-Pacheco J, Kaminski J, et al. Metabolic modeling of single Th17 cells reveals regulators of autoimmunity. Cell. 2021;**184**(16):4168-4185

[4] Puniya BL, Amin R, Lichter B, Moore R, Ciurej A, Bennett SJ, et al. Integrative computational approach identifies drug targets in CD4+ T-cell-mediated immune disorders. npj Systems Biology and Applications. 2021;**7**(1):1-18

[5] Ueno A, Jeffery L, Kobayashi T, Hibi T, Ghosh S, Jijon H. Th17 plasticity and its relevance to inflammatory bowel disease. Journal of Autoimmunity. 2018;**87**:38-49

[6] Ma H, Kang J, Fan W, He H, Huang F. ROR: Nuclear receptor for melatonin or not? Molecules. 2021;**26**(9):2693. DOI: 10.3390/molecules26092693

[7] Capone A, Volpe E. Transcriptional regulators of T helper 17 cell differentiation in health and autoimmune diseases. Frontiers in Immunology. 2020;**11**:348. DOI: 10.3389/fimmu.2020.00348

[8] Karmaus PWF, Chen X, Lim SA, Herrada AA, Nguyen T-LM, Xu B, et al. Metabolic heterogeneity underlies reciprocal fates of TH 17 cell stemness and plasticity. Nature. 2019;**565**(7737):101-105

[9] Bechara R, McGeachy MJ, Gaffen SL. The metabolism-modulating activity of IL-17 signaling in health and disease. The Journal of Experimental Medicine. 2021;**218**(5):e20202191. DOI: 10.1084/jem.20202191

[10] Lee Y, Awasthi A, Yosef N, Quintana FJ, Xiao S, Peters A, et al. Induction and molecular signature of pathogenic TH 17 cells. Nature Immunology. 2012;**13**(10):991-999

[11] Michalek RD, Gerriets VA, Jacobs SR, Macintyre AN, MacIver NJ, Mason EF, et al. Cutting edge: Distinct glycolytic and lipid oxidative metabolic programs are essential for effector and regulatory CD4+ T cell subsets. Journal of Immunology. 2011;**186**(6):3299-3303

[12] Haghikia A, Jörg S, Duscha A, Berg J, Manzel A, Waschbisch A, et al. Dietary fatty acids directly impact central nervous system autoimmunity via the small intestine. Immunity. 2015;**43**(4):817-829

[13] Wang C, Yosef N, Gaublomme J, Wu C, Lee Y, Clish CB, et al. CD5L/AIM regulates lipid biosynthesis and restrains Th17 cell pathogenicity. Cell. 2015;**163**(6):1413-1427

[14] Santori FR, Huang P, Van De Pavert SA, Douglass EF Jr, Leaver DJ, Haubrich BA, et al. Identification of natural RORγ ligands that regulate the development of lymphoid cells. Cell Metabolism. 2015;**21**(2):286-298

[15] Hu X, Wang Y, Hao L-Y, Liu X, Lesch CA, Sanchez BM, et al. Sterol metabolism controls Th 17 differentiation by generating endogenous RORγ agonists. Nature Chemical Biology. 2015;**11**(2):141-147

[16] Soroosh P, Wu J, Xue X, Song J, Sutton SW, Sablad M, et al. Oxysterols are agonist ligands of RORγt and drive Th17 cell differentiation. Proceedings of the National Academy of Sciences. 2014;**111**(33):12163-12168

[17] Bantug GR, Hess C. The burgeoning world of immunometabolites: Th17 cells take center stage. Cell Metabolism. 2017;**26**(4):588-590

[18] Papadopoulou G, Xanthou G. Metabolic rewiring: A new master of Th17 cell plasticity and heterogeneity. The FEBS Journal. Apr 2021. DOI: 10.1111/febs.15853 (Online ahead of print)

[19] CEM G, Armstrong AW, Gudjonsson JE, JNWN B. Psoriasis. Lancet (London, England). 2021;**397**(10281):1301-1315

[20] Ghoreschi K, Balato A, Enerbäck C, Sabat R. Therapeutics targeting the IL-23 and IL-17 pathway in psoriasis. Lancet (London, England). 2021;**397**(10275):754-766

[21] Hao Y, Zhu Y, Zou S, Zhou P, Hu Y, Zhao Q, et al. Metabolic syndrome and psoriasis: Mechanisms and future directions. Frontiers in Immunology. 2021;**12**:711060. DOI: 10.3389/fimmu.2021.711060

[22] Yan D, Blauvelt A, Dey AK, Golpanian RS, Hwang ST, Mehta NN, et al. New frontiers in psoriatic disease research, part II: Comorbidities and targeted therapies. The Journal of Investigative Dermatology. 2021;**141**(10):2328-2337

[23] Boehncke W, Boehncke S, Tobin A, Kirby B. The 'psoriatic march': A concept of how severe psoriasis may drive cardiovascular comorbidity. Experimental Dermatology. 2011;**20**(4):303-307

[24] Choudhary S, Pradhan D, Pandey A, Khan M, Lall R, Ramesh V, et al. The association of metabolic syndrome and psoriasis: A systematic review and meta-analysis of observational study. Endocrine, Metabolic & Immune Disorders—Drug Targets. 2020;**20**(5):703-717

[25] Gottlieb AB, Chao C, Dann F. Psoriasis comorbidities. The Journal of Dermatological Treatment. 2008;**19**(1):5-21

[26] Menter A, Griffiths CEM, Tebbey PW, Horn EJ, Sterry W, Council IP. Exploring the association between cardiovascular and other disease-related risk factors in the psoriasis population: The need for increased understanding across the medical community. Journal of the European Academy of Dermatology and Venereology. 2010;**24**(12):1371-1377

[27] Bajaj S, Mandal S, Singh KG, Prajapati R. Metabolic diseases and associated complications in patients with psoriasis. The Journal of the Association of Physicians of India. 2020;**68**(10):44-46

[28] Bianchi E, Vecellio M, Rogge L. Role of the IL-23/IL-17 pathway in chronic immune-mediated inflammatory diseases: Mechanisms and targeted therapies. Frontiers in Immunology. 2021;**12**:770275. DOI: 10.3389/fimmu.2021.770275

[29] Itoh T, Hatano R, Komiya E, Otsuka H, Narita Y, Aune TM, et al. Biological effects of IL-26 on

T cell–mediated skin inflammation, including psoriasis. The Journal of Investigative Dermatology. 2019;**139**(4):878-889

[30] Wolk K, Witte K, Witte E, Raftery M, Kokolakis G, Philipp S, et al. IL-29 is produced by TH17 cells and mediates the cutaneous antiviral competence in psoriasis. Science Translational Medicine. 2013;**5**(204):204ra129

[31] Krueger JG, Brunner PM. Interleukin-17 alters the biology of many cell types involved in the genesis of psoriasis, systemic inflammation and associated comorbidities. Experimental Dermatology. 2018;**27**(2):115-123

[32] Binger KJ, Côrte-Real BF, Kleinewietfeld M. Immunometabolic regulation of interleukin-17-producing T helper cells: Uncoupling new targets for autoimmunity. Frontiers in Immunology. 2017;**8**:311. DOI: 10.3389/fimmu.2017.00311

[33] Makowski L, Chaib M, Rathmell JC. Immunometabolism: From basic mechanisms to translation. Immunological Reviews. 2020;**295**(1):5-14

[34] Galgani M, Bruzzaniti S, Matarese G. Immunometabolism and autoimmunity. Current Opinion in Immunology. 2020;**67**:10-17

[35] Stathopoulou C, Nikoleri D, Bertsias G. Immunometabolism: An overview and therapeutic prospects in autoimmune diseases. Immunotherapy. 2019;**11**(9):813-829

[36] Man K, Kutyavin VI, Chawla A. Tissue immunometabolism: Development, physiology, and pathobiology. Cell Metabolism. 2017;**25**(1):11-26

[37] Mogilenko DA, Haas JT, L'homme L, Fleury S, Quemener S, Levavasseur M, et al. Metabolic and innate immune cues merge into a specific inflammatory response via the UPR. Cell. 2019;**177**(5):1201-1216

[38] Lercher A, Baazim H, Bergthaler A. Systemic immunometabolism: Challenges and opportunities. Immunity. 2020;**53**(3):496-509

[39] Saravia J, Raynor JL, Chapman NM, Lim SA, Chi H. Signaling networks in immunometabolism. Cell Research. 2020;**30**(4):328-342

[40] Saxton RA, Sabatini DM. mTOR signaling in growth, metabolism, and disease. Cell. 2017;**168**(6):960-976

[41] von Meyenn L, Bertschi NL, Schlapbach C. Targeting T cell metabolism in inflammatory skin disease. Frontiers in Immunology. 2019;**10**:2285. DOI: 10.3389/fimmu.2019.02285

[42] Kelly B, Pearce EL. Amino assets: How amino acids support immunity. Cell Metabolism. 2020;**32**(2):154-175

[43] O'Neill LAJ, Kishton RJ, Rathmell J. A guide to immunometabolism for immunologists. Nature Reviews. Immunology. 2016;**16**(9):553-565

[44] Lin W, Shen P, Song Y, Huang Y, Tu S. Reactive oxygen species in autoimmune cells: Function, differentiation, and metabolism. Frontiers in Immunology. 2021;**12**:635021. DOI: 10.3389/fimmu.2021.635021

[45] Berod L, Friedrich C, Nandan A, Freitag J, Hagemann S, Harmrolfs K, et al. De novo fatty acid synthesis controls the fate between regulatory T and T helper 17 cells. Nature Medicine. 2014;**20**(11):1327-1333

[46] Thomas SP, Denu JM. Short-chain fatty acids activate acetyltransferase

p300. eLife. 2021;**10**:e72171. DOI: 10.7554/eLife.72171

[47] Young KE, Flaherty S, Woodman KM, Sharma-Walia N, Reynolds JM. Fatty acid synthase regulates the pathogenicity of Th17 cells. Journal of Leukocyte Biology. 2017;**102**(5):1229-1235

[48] Cai F, Jin S, Chen G. The effect of lipid metabolism on CD4+ T cells. Mediators of Inflammation. Jan 2021. DOI: 10.1155/2021/6634532

[49] Howie D, Ten Bokum A, Necula AS, Cobbold SP, Waldmann H. The role of lipid metabolism in T lymphocyte differentiation and survival. Frontiers in Immunology. 2018;**8**:1949. DOI: 10.3389/fimmu.2017.01949

[50] Shan J, Jin H, Xu Y. T cell metabolism: A new perspective on Th17/treg cell imbalance in systemic lupus erythematosus. Frontiers in Immunology. 2020;**11**:1027. DOI: 10.3389/fimmu.2020.01027

[51] Dang EV, Barbi J, Yang H-Y, Jinasena D, Yu H, Zheng Y, et al. Control of TH17/Treg balance by hypoxia-inducible factor 1. Cell. 2011;**146**(5):772-784

[52] Gerriets VA, Kishton RJ, Nichols AG, Macintyre AN, Inoue M, Ilkayeva O, et al. Metabolic programming and PDHK1 control CD4+ T cell subsets and inflammation. The Journal of Clinical Investigation. 2015;**125**(1):194-207

[53] Kono M, Yoshida N, Maeda K, Skinner NE, Pan W, Kyttaris VC, et al. Pyruvate dehydrogenase phosphatase catalytic subunit 2 limits Th17 differentiation. Proceedings of the National Academy of Sciences. 2018;**115**(37):9288-9293

[54] Yoshida N, Comte D, Mizui M, Otomo K, Rosetti F, Mayadas TN, et al. ICER is requisite for Th17 differentiation. Nature Communications. 2016;**7**(1):1-13

[55] Xu T, Stewart KM, Wang X, Liu K, Xie M, Ryu JK, et al. Metabolic control of TH 17 and induced T reg cell balance by an epigenetic mechanism. Nature. 2017;**548**(7666):228-233

[56] Roy DG, Chen J, Mamane V, Ma EH, Muhire BM, Sheldon RD, et al. Methionine metabolism shapes T helper cell responses through regulation of epigenetic reprogramming. Cell Metabolism. 2020;**31**(2):250-266

[57] Ladurner A, Schwarz PF, Dirsch VM. Natural products as modulators of retinoic acid receptor-related orphan receptors (RORs). Natural Product Reports. 2021;**38**(4):757-781. DOI: 10.1039/d0np00047g

[58] Shen H, Shi LZ. Metabolic regulation of TH17 cells. Molecular Immunology. 2019;**109**:81-87

[59] Gaublomme JT, Yosef N, Lee Y, Gertner RS, Yang LV, Wu C, et al. Single-cell genomics unveils critical regulators of Th17 cell pathogenicity. Cell. 2015;**163**(6):1400-1412

[60] Tan J, McKenzie C, Potamitis M, Thorburn AN, Mackay CR, Macia L. The role of short-chain fatty acids in health and disease. Advances in Immunology. 2014;**121**:91-119

[61] Lou F, Sun Y, Xu Z, Niu L, Wang Z, Deng S, et al. Excessive polyamine generation in keratinocytes promotes self-RNA sensing by dendritic cells in psoriasis. Immunity. 2020;**53**(1):204-216

[62] Bandyopadhyay M, Larregina AT. Keratinocyte-polyamines and dendritic cells: A bad duet for psoriasis. Immunity. 2020;**53**(1):16-18

[63] Varshney P, Narasimhan A, Mittal S, Malik G, Sardana K, Saini N. Transcriptome profiling unveils the

role of cholesterol in IL-17A signaling in psoriasis. Scientific Reports. 2016;**6**(1):19295. DOI: 10.1038/srep19295

[64] Lebwohl M. Interleukin-23 blockade: Another breakthrough in the treatment of psoriasis. Lancet. 2019;**394**(10198):544-546. DOI: 10.1016/S0140-6736(19)31513-2

[65] Papp KA, Lebwohl MG. Onset of action of biologics in patients with moderate-to-severe psoriasis. Journal of Drugs in Dermatology. 2017;**17**:247-250

[66] Reich K, Gooderham M, Thaçi D, Crowley JJ, Ryan C, Krueger JG, et al. Risankizumab compared with adalimumab in patients with moderate-to-severe plaque psoriasis (IMMvent): A randomised, double-blind, active-comparator-controlled phase 3 trial. Lancet. 2019;**394**(10198):576-586

[67] Jain H, Bhat AR, Dalvi H, Godugu C, Singh SB, Srivastava S. Repurposing approved therapeutics for new indication: Addressing unmet needs in psoriasis treatment. Current Research in Pharmacology and Drug Discovery. 2021;**2**:100041. DOI: 10.1016/j.crphar.2021.100041

[68] Chang JE, Choi MS. A molecular perspective on the potential benefits of metformin for the treatment of inflammatory skin disorders. International Journal of Molecular Sciences. 2020;**21**(23):8960

[69] Naseri M, Hadipour A, Sepaskhah M, Namazi MR. The remarkable beneficial effect of adding oral simvastatin to topical betamethasone for treatment of psoriasis: A double-blind, randomized, placebo-controlled study. Nigerian Journal of Medicine. 2010;**19**(1):58-61

[70] Scheja L, Heeren J. The endocrine function of adipose tissues in health and cardiometabolic disease. Nature Reviews. Endocrinology. 2019;**15**(9):507-524

[71] Winn NC, Cottam MA, Wasserman DH, Hasty AH. Exercise and adipose tissue immunity: Outrunning inflammation. Obesity. 2021;**29**(5):790-801

[72] Wang Q, Wu H. T cells in adipose tissue: Critical players in immunometabolism. Frontiers in Immunology. 2018;**9**:2509. DOI: 10.3389/fimmu.2018.02509

[73] Wang Q, Wang Y, Xu D. The roles of T cells in obese adipose tissue inflammation. Adipocytes. 2021;**10**(1):435-445

[74] Lu J, Zhao J, Meng H, Zhang X. Adipose tissue-resident immune cells in obesity and type 2 diabetes. Frontiers in Immunology. 2019;**10**:1173. DOI: 10.3389/fimmu.2019.01173

[75] Spallanzani RG, Zemmour D, Xiao T, Jayewickreme T, Li C, Bryce PJ, et al. Distinct immunocyte-promoting and adipocyte-generating stromal components coordinate adipose tissue immune and metabolic tenors. Science Immunology. 2019;**4**:eaaw3658. DOI: 10.1126/sciimmunol.aaw3658

[76] Faas M, Ipseiz N, Ackermann J, Culemann S, Grüneboom A, Schröder F, et al. IL-33-induced metabolic reprogramming controls the differentiation of alternatively activated macrophages and the resolution of inflammation. Immunity. 2021;**54**(11):2531-2546

[77] Chen SX, Zhang L-J, Gallo RL. Dermal white adipose tissue: A newly recognized layer of skin innate defense. The Journal of Investigative Dermatology. 2019;**139**(5):1002-1009

[78] Al-Mansoori L, Al-Jaber H, Prince MS, Elrayess MA. Role of

inflammatory cytokines, growth factors and adipokines in adipogenesis and insulin resistance. Inflammation. 2022;**45**(1):31-44

[79] Rijnsburger M, Djuric N, Mulder IA, de Vries HE. Adipokines as immune cell modulators in multiple sclerosis. International Journal of Molecular Sciences. 2021;**22**(19):10845. DOI: 10.3390/ijms221910845

[80] Gerriets VA, Danzaki K, Kishton RJ, Eisner W, Nichols AG, Saucillo DC, et al. Leptin directly promotes T-cell glycolytic metabolism to drive effector T-cell differentiation in a mouse model of autoimmunity. European Journal of Immunology. 2016;**46**(8):1970-1983

[81] Su X, Zhang G, Cheng Y, Wang B. Leptin in skin disease modulation. Clinica Chimica Acta. 2021;**516**:8-14

[82] Su X, Cheng Y, Chang D. The important role of leptin in modulating the risk of dermatological diseases. Frontiers in Immunology. 2021;**11**: 593564. DOI: 10.3389/fimmu.2020.593564

[83] Li Y, Yang Q, Cai D, Guo H, Fang J, Cui H, et al. Resistin, a novel host defense peptide of innate immunity. Frontiers in Immunology. 2021;**12**:699807. DOI: 10.3389/fimmu.2021.699807

[84] Lee M-J, Wu Y, Fried SK. Adipose tissue remodeling in pathophysiology of obesity. Current Opinion in Clinical Nutrition and Metabolic Care. 2010;**13**(4):371-376

[85] Langan SM, Seminara NM, Shin DB, Troxel AB, Kimmel SE, Mehta NN, et al. Prevalence of metabolic syndrome in patients with psoriasis: A population-based study in the United Kingdom. The Journal of Investigative Dermatology. 2012;**132**(3):556-562

[86] Warren RB, Marsden A, Tomenson B, Mason KJ, Soliman MM, Burden AD, et al. Identifying demographic, social and clinical predictors of biologic therapy effectiveness in psoriasis: A multicentre longitudinal cohort study. The British Journal of Dermatology. 2019;**180**(5):1069-1076

[87] Aune D, Snekvik I, Schlesinger S, Norat T, Riboli E, Vatten LJ. Body mass index, abdominal fatness, weight gain and the risk of psoriasis: A systematic review and dose–response meta-analysis of prospective studies. European Journal of Epidemiology. 2018;**33**(12):1163-1178

[88] Hwang J, Yoo JA, Yoon H, Han T, Yoon J, An S, et al. The role of leptin in the association between obesity and psoriasis. Biomolecules & Therapeutics. 2021;**29**(1):11-21

[89] Dopytalska K, Baranowska-Bik A, Roszkiewicz M, Bik W, Walecka I. The role of leptin in selected skin diseases. Lipids in Health and Disease. 2020;**19**(1):1-10

[90] Yamazaki F. Psoriasis: Comorbidities. The Journal of Dermatology. 2021;**48**(6):732-740

[91] Ruiyang B, Panayi A, Ruifang W, Peng Z, Siqi F. Adiponectin in psoriasis and its comorbidities: A review. Lipids in Health and Disease. 2021;**20**(1):1-11

[92] Shibata S, Tada Y, Hau CS, Mitsui A, Kamata M, Asano Y, et al. Adiponectin regulates psoriasiform skin inflammation by suppressing IL-17 production from γδ-T cells. Nature Communications. 2015;**6**(1):1-14

[93] Surendar J, Frohberger SJ, Karunakaran I, Schmitt V, Stamminger W, Neumann A-L, et al. Adiponectin limits IFN-γ and IL-17 producing CD4 T cells in obesity by restraining cell

intrinsic glycolysis. Frontiers in Immunology. 2019;**10**:2555. DOI: 10.3389/fimmu.2019.02555

[94] Michelet X, Dyck L, Hogan A, Loftus RM, Duquette D, Wei K, et al. Metabolic reprogramming of natural killer cells in obesity limits antitumor responses. Nature Immunology. 2018;**19**(12):1330-1340

[95] Koussiouris J, Looby N, Anderson M, Kulasingam V, Chandran V. Metabolomics studies in psoriatic disease: A review. Metabolites. 2021;**11**(6):375. DOI: 10.3390/metabo11060375

[96] Sorokin AV, Domenichiello AF, Dey AK, Yuan Z-X, Goyal A, Rose SM, et al. Bioactive lipid mediator profiles in human psoriasis skin and blood. The Journal of Investigative Dermatology. 2018;**138**(7):1518-1528

[97] Sorokin AV, Norris PC, English JT, Dey AK, Chaturvedi A, Baumer Y, et al. Identification of proresolving and inflammatory lipid mediators in human psoriasis. Journal of Clinical Lipidology. 2018;**12**(4):1047-1060

[98] Dutkiewicz EP, Hsieh K-T, Urban PL, Chiu H-Y. Temporal correlations of skin and blood metabolites with clinical outcomes of biologic therapy in psoriasis. Journal of Applied Laboratory Medicine. 2020;**5**(5):877-888

[99] Tarentini E, Odorici G, Righi V, Paganelli A, Giacomelli L, Mirisola V, et al. Integrated metabolomic analysis and cytokine profiling define clusters of immuno-metabolic correlation in new-onset psoriasis. Scientific Reports. 2021;**11**(1):1-12

[100] Lynch SV, Pedersen O. The human intestinal microbiome in health and disease. The New England Journal of Medicine. 2016;**375**(24):2369-2379

[101] Chen L, Li J, Zhu W, Kuang Y, Liu T, Zhang W, et al. Skin and gut microbiome in psoriasis: Gaining insight into the pathophysiology of it and finding novel therapeutic strategies. Frontiers in Microbiology. 2020;**11**:589726. DOI: 10.3389/fmicb.2020.589726

[102] Aydin B, Arga KY, Karadag AS. Omics-driven biomarkers of psoriasis: Recent insights, current challenges, and future prospects. Clinical, Cosmetic and Investigational Dermatology. 2020;**13**:611-625. DOI: 10.2147/CCID.S227896

[103] Liu Y, Cui S, Sun J, Yan X, Han D. Identification of potential biomarkers for psoriasis by DNA methylation and gene expression datasets. Frontiers in Genetics. 2021;**12**:722803. DOI: h10.3389/fgene.2021.722803

[104] Su W, Wei Y, Huang B, Ji J. Identification of hub genes and immune infiltration in psoriasis by bioinformatics method. Frontiers in Genetics. 2021;**12**:606065. DOI: 10.3389/fgene.2021.606065

Chapter 5

Immune Markers in Psoriasis

Mihaela Surcel, Adriana Narcisa Munteanu,
Carolina Constantin and Monica Neagu

Abstract

Psoriasis is a chronic inflammatory skin disorder with high immunological background caused by a complex interplay between an altered immune system, genetic factors, autoantigens, lifestyle, and environmental factors. Extensive literature in recent years highlighted the crucial role played by the immune system in the pathogenesis of this pathology. Although it is unequivocally accepted that psoriasis is a T-cell mediated autoimmune condition, both innate and specific immune cells are highly involved in the pathogenesis of psoriasis. The aberrant interactions between immune cells and resident hyper-proliferative keratinocytes are mediated by immune and non-immune related molecules which lead to amplification of the local immune responses, that maintain the chronic inflammatory status. In this chapter, we will highlight the immune molecules resident in the psoriatic tissue or appending to the blood circulation that can indicate the prognosis of this systemic autoimmune disease. Moreover, we will focus on immune cells resident or circulating ones that can pin-point the clinical evolution of the psoriatic disease. All these data can be developed in immune markers patterns that aid psoriasis diagnosis and/or future (immune) therapies.

Keywords: psoriasis, autoimmunity, inflammation, immune markers, cytokines

1. Introduction

Psoriasis (Ps) is a chronic inflammatory T-cell mediated disease, that is manifested mainly as skin lesions and extracutaneous comorbidities, the overall symptomatology of the disease having a strong impact on the patients' life quality [1].

Worldwide, the prevalence of this disease is increasing for both adults and children, and varies between 0.09% and 11.4%, respectively between 1.5% and 5% in most developed countries. The disease incidence depends on age, sex, ethnicity, geographical regions, and environmental factors [2]. Ps especially affects Caucasians as compared to other ethnic groups and is more common in high-income countries. In children, the incidence increases with age, the median age at diagnosis being 10.6 years, with a higher prevalence in girls compared to boys [3].

The exact causes of Ps onset are still unknown. Ps is a complex and multifactorial skin condition that occurs on an altered genetic and immunologic background, favored by environmental factors [4] and aggravated by extrinsic risk factors and intrinsic risk factors [5].

Its complexity rides also on the fact that Ps presents a wide spectrum of skin lesions therefore, the specific clinical type of Ps is important in choosing the adequate treatment protocol. Ps is histologically characterized by keratinocytes (KCs) hyper-proliferation which induces acanthosis, elongation of the rete ridges, hyperkeratosis, and parakeratosis, and an inflammatory infiltrate consisting mainly of dendritic cells (DCs) and T cells [6].

For many years, Ps was classified as an immune-mediated inflammatory disorder and less as an autoimmune condition due to the fact that the autoantigens causing T cell activation remain unknown. Recent studies reported the identification of four possible autoantigens involved in Ps' pathogenesis: KCs – derived antimicrobial peptide LL-37 (cathelicidin) [7], ADAMTS-like-protein 5 (a disintegrin- and metal-loprotease domain-containing thrombospondin type 1 motif-like 5) produced by melanocytes, lipid antigens generated by phospholipase A2 group IVD (PLA2G4D) [8] and keratin 17 derived from hair follicles [9]. Studies regarding the autoimmune character of Ps have also focused on the existence of specific autoantibodies, the most common being anti-stratum corneum antibodies [10] and anti-heat shock protein 65 [11]. However, the clinical significance of these autoantibodies remains still evasive.

Although Ps is recognized as one of the most prevalent T-cell mediated chronic inflammatory skin conditions, its pathogenesis involved both innate and adaptive immune cells. Pathogenic crosstalk between hyper-proliferative resident KCs and immune cells mediated by immune and non-immune molecules are responsible for the development and maintenance of Ps' inflammatory state [12].

Two phases were described in the Ps' pathogenesis: initiation of psoriatic events, in which the cells belonging to the innate immunity (DCs, NK cells, Mϕ-macrophages) play an important role, and the phase of maintaining inflammatory status, in which the key players belong to the adaptive immunity (T helper (h)-cell subsets). In earlier stages of the disease, under the action of triggering factors (genetic, environmental, physical injury, infections, stress), KCs and cells belonging to innate immunity (plasmacytoid (P) DCs, NK cells, Mϕ) produce tumor necrosis factor (TNF)-α, interferon (IFN)-α, IFN-β, IFN-γ, interleukin (IL)-1β, IL-6 thus activating the myeloid (M)DCs. In the initiation of psoriatic events, a starting key is represented by the activation of PDCs, secreting two type I IFNs (IFN-α, IFN-β), further promoting MDCs activation. Activated MDCs, by secreting IL-12 and IL-23, will determine the differentiation of naïve T-cells into Th1, Th17, and Th22 subpopulations. TNF-α, IFN-γ, IL-17, and IL-22 secreted by these effector subsets, will be able to activate KCs, which will produce a variety of cytokines (TNF-α, IL-1β, IL-6, IL-8, IL-19, IL-36), chemokines (CXCL1/2/3/5/8), antimicrobial peptides (LL-37) and S100 proteins, thus propagating and maintaining the inflammatory status [13–15]. A general outline of the initiation and propagation stages of Ps is depicted in **Figure 1**.

Ps in not only a skin disease, it also has significant disabling systemic manifestations [13]. The disease is frequently associated with arthritic, metabolic, cardiovascular, and psychological comorbidities, which can lead to increased mortality among affected persons [16]. Knowing and understanding the relationship between Ps and other associated pathologies is particularly important for optimal clinical management of patients.

Depending on the Ps severity, there is a wide range of therapeutic options, from the traditional topical treatment, phototherapy, and systemic treatments, to new biological therapies. Despite various treatment options available, Ps still remains an incurable and undertreated disease [17], and finding an adjuvant treatment [18] to help existing ones remains a challenge for researchers.

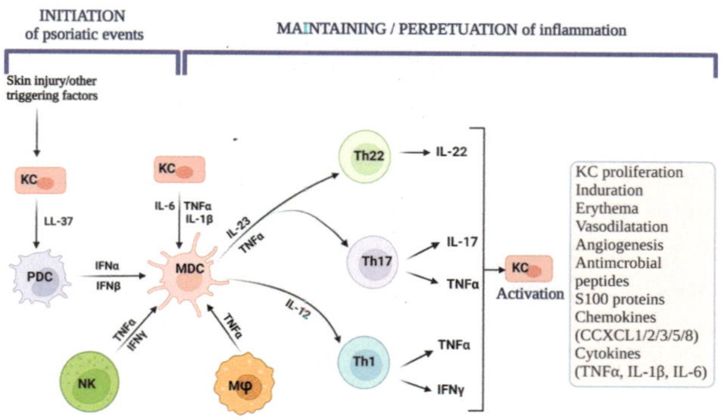

Figure 1.
Immune mechanisms are associated with the onset of psoriatic events and the maintenance of the inflammatory status. KCs and innate immune cells are activated by triggers that secrete cytokines, leading to the differentiation in Th1, Th17, and Th22 cells via IL-12, IL-23, and TNF-α secreted by activated MDCs. These effectors promote KCs activation through TNF-α, IFN-γ, IL17, and IL22, leading to the perpetuation of the inflammatory cycle by generating AMP (LL-37, β-defensins, S100 proteins) and by secreting of cytokines (TNF-α, IL-6, IL-1β) and chemokines (CXCL1, CXCL2, CXCL3, CXCL5, CXCL8, CXCL9, CXCL10, CXCL20). Created with BioRender.com.

Although it is unequivocally accepted that Ps is a T-cell mediated condition, both innate and specific immune cells are highly involved in the pathogenesis of Ps. The aberrant interactions between immune cells and resident hyper-proliferative KCs are mediated by immune and non-immune related molecules which lead to amplification of the local immune responses, that maintain the chronic inflammatory status. In this chapter, we will highlight the immune molecules resident in the psoriatic tissue or appending to the blood circulation that can indicate the prognosis of this systemic autoimmune disease. Moreover, we will focus on immune cells resident or circulating ones that can pinpoint the clinical evolution of the psoriatic disease. All these data can be developed in immune markers patterns that aid Ps' diagnosis and/or future (immune)therapies development.

2. Immune cells in the development of psoriasis

As already stated, Ps is an immune-mediated inflammatory skin disorder based on the pathological crosstalk between KCs and immune cells sustained by a complex array of pro-inflammatory cytokines/chemokines. Disturbances in both innate and adaptive immune responses, as well as hyper-proliferative KCs, have important roles in triggering the early psoriatic events and in sustaining the chronic inflammation that follows. Immune cells are highly involved in both phases of Ps pathogenesis: innate immune cells (PDCs, MDCs, NK cells, Mϕ, neutrophils) play a major role in the initiation of the psoriatic events, while adaptive immune cells (Th-cell subsets: Th17, Th22, Th1) are the main actors in maintaining the inflammatory status of the disease.

2.1 Tissue resident immune cells

Dendritic cells, professional antigen-presenting cells (APCs), are crucial in the early stages of the disease due to their ability to recognize the antimicrobial peptides (AMP) (LL-37, β-defensins, S100 proteins) released by damaged KCs in response to various triggering factors [19]. LL-37, recognized as an autoantigen in Ps, binds to self-DNA and RNA from other damaged cells and stimulates toll-like receptor (TLR) 9, respectively TLR8 in PDCs. Activated PDCs will secrete IFN-α thus promoting MDCs activation. These activated cells will migrate into draining lymph nodes and by secreting high amounts of IL-12, IL-23 and TNF-α will further guide the differentiation of naïve T-cells in Th1, Th17, and Th22 populations [15]. These effector subsets will produce TNF-α, IFN-α, IL-17, IL-22 thus promoting KCs proliferation. Activated KCs will perpetuate the inflammatory cycle by generating AMP (LL-37, β-defensins, S100 proteins) and by secreting cytokines (TNF-α, IL-6, IL-1β) and chemokines (CXCL1, CXCL2, CXCL3, CXCL5, CXCL8, CXCL9, CXCL10, CXCL20) [14]. LL-37 secreted by KCs will be recognized by LL-37-activated PDCs which will perpetuate the pathogenic mechanism. IL-17, CXCL1, CXCL2, and CXCL8 released by Th17 and KCs mediate the recruitment of neutrophils which will migrate to the psoriatic lesions, release large amounts of reactive oxygen species (ROS), granules and form neutrophil extracellular traps (NETs) [20].

MDCs can be also PDCs-independent activated, by CCL20 released by KCs in response to the skin microbiome, drugs, and injury [21]. Once activated, MDCs will initiate the inflammatory state in Ps. Two subpopulations of dermal MDCs have been described in psoriatic lesions: $CD11c^{+}BDCA\text{-}1^{+}$ cells, which are also found in normal skin, and $CD11c^{+}BDCA\text{-}1^{-}$ cells, characterized by the ability to produce inflammatory cytokines. $CD11c^{+}BDCA\text{-}1^{+}$ cells are comparable in number to those found in normal skin, while $CD11c^{+}BDCA\text{-}1^{-}$ cells, named "inflammatory MDCs", are increased 30-fold in psoriatic lesions. Both subpopulations of MDCs induce T cell proliferation and cause differentiation into Th1 cells. In addition, inflammatory MDCs are responsible for the IL-23-induced Th17 stimulation [22].

Neutrophils, important representatives of innate immune cells, are considered to be regulators between innate and adaptive immune systems. Neutrophils are attracted to the psoriatic plaque by chemokines (CXCL1, CXCL2) and cytokines (IL-8) released by activated KCs, forming Munro microabscesses, an important histopathological feature of Ps [23]. Respiratory burst, degranulation, and NETs formation, the main offensive function of neutrophils, are correlated with Ps' development and progression.

During activation, neutrophils mobilize and release granular components thus inducing their own migration and activating their antimicrobial activities. NE (neutrophil elastase), MPO (myeloperoxidase), and LL-37 (recognized as an autoantigen in Ps) were reported to be highly involved in Ps. NE and cathepsin G activate IL-36 leading to an exacerbated tissue inflammation [24]. In Ps patients' circulatory neutrophils have increased MPO and NOX2 (reduced nicotinamide adenine dinucleotide phosphate-NADPH oxidase) activities and enhanced respiratory burst, releasing more ROS compared to healthy individuals [25]. Overproduction of ROS induces proliferation and differentiation of Th1, Th17, and Th22 cells, and inhibits regulatory T cells (Tregs). Inflammatory cytokines secreted by these T cell subsets along with VEGF, stimulate KCs proliferation and angiogenesis [26, 27]. In psoriatic plaque and pustules, NETs are overexpressed and IL-17 releasing cells will be activated. Accordingly, the synthesis of inflammatory mediators will be stimulated, leading to auto-amplification of neutrophil's overall activities [20]. Inhibition of neutrophils degranulation and suppression of respiratory burst can become new therapeutical targets for alleviating Ps symptoms.

Macrophages, cells with phagocytic and antigen-presenting properties, are important innate immune sentinels. Mϕ is abundant in psoriatic lesions and are involved in the inflammatory process due to their ability to produce cytokines and inflammatory mediators. The most representative monokines are IL-23, responsible for the differentiation of Th17 [28], and TNF-α responsible for Th22 differentiation [29].

NK cells, recognized for their ability to kill virally infected cells and cancer cells, appear to be involved in the pathogenesis of Ps, but their role still remains controversial. Thus, Ottaviani et al. identified a subpopulation of NK cells with the $CD56^{bright}CD16^{-}CD158^{+}$ phenotype able to produce large amounts of IFN-γ, and these cells are recruited by KC activated through chemokine secretion (CXCL10, CCL5) [30]. Thus recruited, NK cells can contribute to the inflammatory environment of the skin. On the other hand, Dunphy et al. noted the presence of NK cells in skin lesions of Ps patients, but these cells were characterized by poor degranulation potency and reduced secretion of proinflammatory cytokines (IFN-γ and TNF-α) [31].

NKT cells are a distinct cellular subset that exhibits both T-cell receptor (TCR) and NK cells lineage markers and can produce large amounts of cytokines in response to various stimuli, such as lipids and cytokines. NKT cells have been identified in psoriatic lesions and were reported a decreased following treatment [32]. Bonish et al. have shown that NKT cells ($CD161^{+}$) can produce large amounts of IFN-γ that induce CD1d overexpression on KCs in psoriatic lesions. These KCs subsequently activate NKT cells to produce IFN-γ. Bonish et al. also suggested that the interactions between NKT and KCs could provide a relevant mechanism in the pathogenesis of Ps [33]. Several NKT cells can secrete IL-17 and IL-22 after IL-1β and IL-23 stimulation. These cells, named NKT17, express high levels of RORγT, and were found in the lung, liver, marginal lymph nodes, and skin [34], but their role in the skin is not yet well defined.

Other innate immune cells involved in Ps pathogenesis are innate lymphoid cells (ILCs) and γδT cells, which are activated in Ps and may represent important sources of Il-22 and IL-17.

ILCs are members of lymphoid lineage and are involved in the early response to infections in the skin, lung, and gastrointestinal tract. In the absence of an antigen-specific receptor, they are activated through signals from cytokine and NK receptors and secrete high levels of cytokines. Within the three types of known ILCs, ILC3 type seems to be involved in Ps due to its ability to produce IL-17 and IL-22. Depending on the presence or absence of natural cytotoxicity receptor (NCR), ILC3 were classified into NCR+ILC3 (increased in psoriatic lesions), NCR^{-}ILC3 (commonly in normal skin), and lymphoid tissue inducer cells (LTi). When they are activated, NCR^{+}ILC3 secrete IL-22, NCR-ILC3 produce IL-17, IL-22 and IFN-γ, LTi-lymphotoxin, IL-17, and IL-22 [35]. Vilanova et al. reported an increased amount of IL-22 and IL-17 producing ILC3 in psoriatic skin, correlated with disease severity [36]. Another study showed that NCR^{+}ILC3 isolated from psoriatic skin, stimulated by IL-2, IL-23, and IL-1β, produce large amounts of IL-22, but not IL-17 [37], thus suggesting that ILC3 contribute to the development of Ps via IL-22.

γδT cells are involved in the pathology of allergic and autoimmune diseases in mice and humans and contribute to the development of Ps by IL-17 production. Unlike αβT cells, γδT cells express TCR that consists of γ and δ chains. They interact with both innate and adaptive immune cells, and with non-immune tissue cells, and can promote tissue repair and wound healing [38]. γδT cells are able to recruit inflammatory myeloid cells and modulate classical T cells functions by increasing Th17 inflammatory responses and/or by reducing the activity of Treg cells [39]. In addition to IL-17, they also secrete IFN-γ, IL-22, and GM-CSF. Cai et al. reported that both human and murine dermal innate γδT cells are an important source of IL-17 in the skin upon IL-23 stimulation, and may represent a novel target for the Ps' treatment [40].

However, recent studies have shown that γδT cells account for up to 1% of T cells in Ps, the majority of IL-17-producing T cells being αβT cells and not γδT emphasizing that human Ps is mainly driven by αβT cells [41]. However, more studies are needed to accurately determine the involvement of γδT cells in Ps.

T lymphocytes, cellular exponents of the adaptive immune system, are the key players in the phase of maintaining the inflammatory status in Ps. The pathogenic interactions between T-cells subsets (T-CD8$^+$, autoreactive T cells Th1, Th17, Th22,), DCs, and KCs, result in a self-maintaining inflammatory status with TNFα/IL-23/IL17 axis as a key point [42]. Although the involvement of T cells in Ps has been extensively studied, the gradual scaling of T-cell mediated events is not yet fully elucidated. Casciano et al. pointed out the four T-dependent stages consisting of a skin T cell activation phase, the onset of chronic inflammation, the maintenance of the inflammatory status, and the migration of specific subsets of T cells outside the skin possibly involved in Ps extra-cutaneous manifestations [43]. Various T cell sub-populations have been recognized as involved in Ps pathogenesis.

T-CD8 cells have a crucial role in Ps plaque formation and strongly sustain the autoimmune nature of the disease. DCs recognize and present epidermal autoantigens (LL-37, ADAMTS-like-protein 5, keratin 17) to IL-17-producing T-CD8 cells, in an MHC-restricted manner. Human leukocyte antigen (HLA)-C*06:02, a specific MHC allele is involved in the autoimmune T-cell response in Ps [44]. Recent studies have shown that T-CD8 cells accumulate in active and resolved psoriatic lesions as tissue-resident memory T cells (TRM) with αβTCR [41] and have an IFN-γ/IL-17/IL-22 cytokine profile (thus maintaining the inflammatory status) [45]. Autoantigens recognition by Tc1/Tc17 cells induces the secretion of cytokines that will cause the onset of KCs hyper-proliferation. Activated KCs will contribute to the propagation and maintenance of inflammation through the secretion of antimicrobial peptides, cytokines, and chemokines [46].

Activated DCs also secrete IL-12 and IL-23, inducing the differentiation in Th1 and Th17 subsets of naive T lymphocytes. In response, these effector subsets will produce TNF-α, IFN-α, IL-17, IL-22 thus promoting KCs proliferation.

Initially, Ps was considered a predominantly Th1-mediated disease, being reported as an imbalance between Th1 and Th2 cells. This imbalance was due to the increasing of IFN-γ expressions as compared to low levels obtained for IL-4, IL-5, or IL-10, which are specific Th2 cytokines [47]. Th1 cells, a subset of T-CD4+ cells, are defined by activation of transcription factors STAT4 and T-bet and the secretion of proinflammatory cytokines (IFN-γ, IL-2, and TNF). Th1 cells and IFN-γ levels were found elevated in psoriatic lesions [48]. IFN-γ, along with TNF-α, IFN-α, IFN-β, IL-1β, and IL-6 activate IL-12 and IL-23 – producing MDCs in the initial phase of the disease, and under the influence of Th1 cells, KCs secrete pro-inflammatory mediators (IL-1β and IL-18) that are further involved in the differentiation of Th1 and Th17 cells [49]. Although the involvement of IFN-γ-producing Th1 cells has been extensively studied, the results of clinical trials based on anti-IFN-γ antibodies did not have the expected results [50].

Extensive literature in recent years has proven the clinical efficacy of IL-17 inhibitors, highlighting the important role of IL-17-secreting lymphocytes—Th17 and Tc17 cells—in Ps. Th17 cells are a T-CD4+ subset defined by mainly IL-17A, IL-17F, IL-22, IL-21, and IL-26 secretion, and express retinoic acid receptor-related orphan receptor-γt (ROR-γt) and IL-23 receptor (R) [51]. Th17-derived proinflammatory cytokines have a critical role in the pathogenesis of many autoimmune and inflammatory diseases, including Ps. Th17 cells activated by IL-1β and IL-23, trigger inflammation and autoimmunity, while activation through IL-6 and transforming growth factor (TGF)-β is involved in tissue defense and homeostasis [52]. Although NK and γδT cells also synthesize IL-17, Th17 remains the main source of IL-17.

IL-12 and IL-23 secreted by activated MDCs cause differentiation into Th1, Th17, and Th22 effector cells. IL-23 secreted by MDCs induces the differentiation of Th17 cells, and by activation of IL-23R expressed on Th17 cell, maintain the local inflammation [53]. IL-17A released by Th17 cells will promote the KCs activation, which will maintain the chronic inflammatory status through the secretion of antimicrobial peptides, cytokines, and chemokines. Activated Th17 cells are present in psoriatic lesions [54], and elevated levels of IL-23, a Th17-driving cytokine, were reported in lesional skin [55]. These data sustain the importance of IL-23/T17 axis in the development of Ps.

Although it is recognized that Th17 cells play a critical role in the Ps pathogenesis, and the secreted cytokines are strongly involved not only in the onset and development of the disease but can cause complications of other associated diseases, more research is needed regarding the pathogenicity of Th17 cells in Ps.

Another subset of T-$CD4^+$ lymphocytes involved in Ps pathogenesis is represented by Th22 cells. Th22 differentiate from naive T cells in the presence of IL-23, IL-6, and TNF-α, and upon activation, these cells will produce IL-22, TNF-α, IL-13, and IL-26, but not IFN-γ or IL-17. IL-22 can induce specific chemokines that will increase specific effector responses mediated by the IL-23 / Th17 axis [56], the network leading to epidermal hyperplasia and hypergranulosis. In a recent study, Cheuk et al. demonstrated that epidermal Th22 and Tc17 cells are retained in healed psoriatic skin and can induce the recurrence of the disease in previously affected areas through the secretion of specific cytokines [57].

Another significant role in Ps' pathogenesis is played by Tregs lymphocytes, cells that suppress the autoimmune responses and other aberrant or excessive immune responses against non-self-antigens [58]. Tregs play an important role in maintaining homeostasis and can cause local suppression of the activity of other immune cells, including Th1 and Th17 cells. In Ps, the suppressive function of Tregs is altered, resulting in a Th17/Tregs imbalance and an upregulation of pro-inflammatory cytokines [59]. The decreased suppression function of Tregs can be a result of elevated levels of IL-6 produced by DCs, Th17, and endothelial cells, which inhibit per se Tregs' activity. Furthermore, Tregs cells can differentiate into a Th17 phenotype in Ps. $IL\text{-}17A^+Foxp3^+CD4^+$ cells were found in psoriatic lesions from patients with severe Ps, thus highlighting Tregs' potential to differentiate into an IL-17A-producing phenotype [60]. Thus, in Ps Tregs behave in a Th17 cells manner and hence are unable to exert their suppressor functions. Nussbaum et al. suggested several ways of restoring Th17/Tregs balance: induction of Tregs (using anti-TNF-α, folic acid analogs, phototherapy, vitamin D, retinoids, anti-IL-17, and anti-IL-23), downregulation of Th17 cells (using phototherapy, folic acid analogs, retinoids, and anti-IL-17) and inhibition of Tregs plasticity (using pan-PKCs inhibitor and anti-IL-23) [59].Although the involvement of B lymphocytes in Ps pathogenesis has been not as much studied compared to T lymphocytes, recent years' research has highlighted the possible role of IL-10-secreting regulatory B cells (Bregs) in disease's attenuation. Bregs are a subset with regulatory properties exerted mainly by the production of cytokines like IL-10, TGF-β. These subpopulations are associated with the regulation and control of excessive inflammatory responses. Recently was underlined the heterogeneity of Bregs cells, suggests that this population may develop from any subset of B cells in the context of adequate stimulation [61]. IL-10-secreting B cells seem to have an inhibitory effect in Ps development. Thus, Yanaba et al. have shown that Bregs cells suppress Ps-like skin inflammation induced by imiquimod (IMQ), a potent agonist for TLR7 and – 8 in a murine experimental model [62]. Although recombinant IL-10 was one of the first biologic agents used in Ps, the clinical trials have not been completed to be introduced in the clinical management of Ps patients, thus more studies are needed to determine Bregs involvement in the course of Ps.

2.2 Circulatory immune cells

Although the distribution of peripheral blood cell populations can be a valuable indicator for establishing the patient's immune status and ability to develop an effective defense against pathogenic factors, circulatory immune cells have been less studied in Ps as compared to tissue-resident immune cells. Due to their important role in the pathogenesis of Ps, lymphocyte populations and subpopulations have been the most studied circulating immune cells. Tissue immune cells are mirrored by the circulatory ones as there is a constant circulation between these sites (**Figure 2**).

In the peripheral blood of Ps' patients, an increased T-$CD4^+$ cells activation and an imbalance in the Th1/Th2 ratio, with high Th1 and low Th2 phenotypes have been reported [63]. Also, higher levels of IFN-γ, IL-2, and IL-10, decreased concentration of IL-4, and increased expression of T-bet mRNA (Th1-specific transcription factor) sustain that Ps is predominantly a Th1-mediated disease [64]. In the early stages of Ps, the patients have increased IFN-γ expression, while patients in the chronic stage have high levels of IL-10. All these findings suggest a possible shift from Th1 to Th2 response in order to down-regulate the inflammatory response [65].

In a recent study regarding the immunophenotyping of T cells in Ps' peripheral blood, increased Th1/Th17 cells and decreased Th2/Tregs cells were reported. The percentages

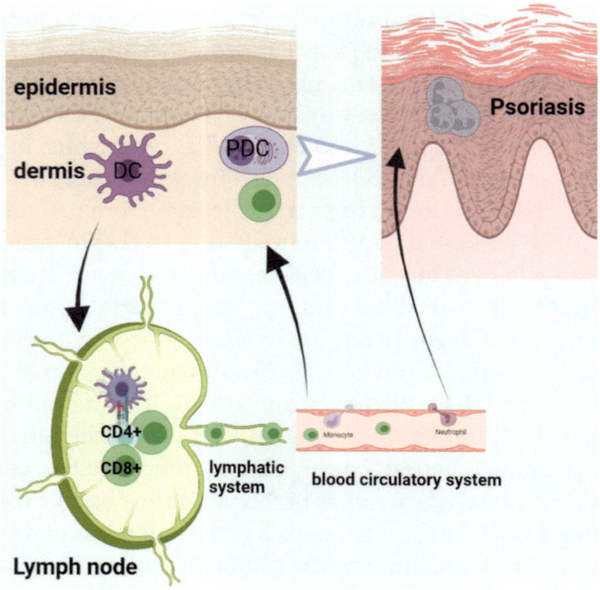

Figure 2.
Immune cells like activated dermal DCs can circulate through the lymphatic system into lymph nodes where DCs activate various T cell subpopulations that can travel into the skin and contribute to the activation of PDCs; the activation of cells within the skin would trigger the chemotaxis of monocytes and neutrophils into the skin and increase the inflammatory status of the psoriatic lesion. Created with BioRender.com.

of Th1/Th17 cells were positively correlated with disease severity (PASI score) [63]. A positive correlation has also been reported between elevated levels of IL-21$^+$ Th17 cells and IL-21 found in peripheral blood of Ps patients with the severity of the disease. The study also has shown that IL-21 can promote the differentiation into the Th17 subset, and recommends IL-21 as a potential immune marker [66].

Another T-CD4$^+$ cell subset involved in Ps' pathogenesis is Th22. Luan et al. reported elevated levels of circulating Th22, Tc22, and IL-22 in patients showing a positive correlation between Th22, IL-22, and PASI score. Nevertheless, no correlation was observed between circulating Tc22 and PASI score [67].

The studies regarding Tregs cells distribution in peripheral blood are controversial. Thus, some authors report a low frequency of circulating Tregs in Ps [68], others observed high percentages of Tregs correlated with PASI scores in moderate to severe Ps [69], and others show no differences compared to healthy volunteers [70]. Although the relevance of Tregs distribution in the periphery remains unclear, the decreased suppressive function and an altered Th17/Tregs balance contribute to the exacerbation of Ps.

T follicular helper (Tfh) cells are a specialized subset of T-CD4+ cells expressing increased levels of CXCR5, inducible T cell costimulatory (ICOS), programmed death protein-1 (PD-1), and the transcription factors B cell lymphoma 6 (Bcl-6). This sub-population actively secrets high levels of IL-21, IL-17, and IFN-γ [71]. Tfh cells are activated in Ps and identifying a higher percentage of circulating Tfh17 (CXCR3-CCR6+ phenotype) correlates with disease' severity. Thus, the frequency of circulating Tfh cells and the secretion of cytokines are significantly decreased after one month of treatment. All these findings indicate that activated circulating Tfh cells are involved in Ps pathogenesis and can constitute a potential therapeutic target for psoriatic disease [72].

In contrast to T-CD4$^+$ cells, considered the key subset of pathogenic T lymphocytes, circulating T-CD8$^+$ cells have been less studied and characterized. The frequency of circulating T-CD8$^+$ cells which express cutaneous lymphocyte antigen (CLA) is higher in Ps patients compared to healthy individuals and is strongly correlated with PASI score [73]. Colombo et al. evaluated circulating IL17$^+$/IFN-γ^+/IL-17/IL-22$^+$ T-CD8 cells in Ps, psoriatic arthritis (PsA), and rheumatoid arthritis (RA), and reported high levels of IFN-γ^+T-CD8 cells in PsA compared to Ps. A significant correlation between the extent and severity of Ps and the frequency of circulating IL-17$^+$T-CD8 cells was as well reported [74].

Although B cells play also an important role in skin inflammation, their distribution in peripheral blood has been poorly studied in Ps. Lu et al. found upregulated percentages of CD19$^+$ B cells in peripheral blood mononuclear cells (PBMCs) of Ps patients, which were positively correlated with PASI score. The authors also investigated the expression of CD40, CD44, CD80, CD86, and CD11b on B cells in 4 clinical types of Ps and showed that the expressions of these activation markers are different in various types of Ps [75]. Other studies reported decreased circulating IL-10-producing Bregs cells in Ps, negatively correlated with Th1, Th17 cells, and IFNγ^+ and IL-17$^+$ NKT cells. During apremilast treatment, these values increased and were correlated with the clinical response [76, 77].

NK cells, known for their anti-viral and anti-tumoral functions, were found in the inflammatory infiltrate of the psoriatic lesions. Even though Ps is a skin disorder, there have been reported changes in circulating NK cells. The number of circulating NK cells is reduced in Ps patients. The levels of circulating IFN-γ and TNF-α are similar to healthy controls [78]. The low levels of NK cells in Ps patients peripheral blood, correlated with a lower frequency of cells expressing NK specific markers (CD56, CD16, CD94, CD158a) but no correlation with the severity of the disease [79]. NK cells had increased expression of the apoptosis-associated Fas receptor and lower expression of CD94 and NKG2A. In addition to its ability to induce apoptosis, Fas receptor is also able to induce the production of proinflammatory cytokines, including TNF-α, a key cytokine in Ps. No differences between Ps patients and controls were reported for $CD56^{dim}CD16^{+}$ and $CD56^{bright}CD16^{-}$ in peripheral blood [80]. Significantly decreased circulating $CD3^{-}CD16^{+}CD56^{+}$ NK cells correlated with increased B lymphocytes in Ps patients were also reported [81]. The role of circulating NK cells in Ps pathogenesis remains still unclear and a subject for further investigation.

In our studies, we identified several phenotypic changes in lymphocyte main populations in the IMQ-mice model. We reported decreased percentages of circulating $T\text{-}CD4^{+}$ and $B\text{-}CD19^{+}$ cells, and elevated levels of $T\text{-}CD8^{+}$ and $NK1.1^{+}$ cells in IMQ-treated mice as compared to healthy animals [82]. For NK cells phenotypic characterization we used a large panel of surface markers including activation, maturation, and markers for cytokine receptors. The results showed important differences in IMQ-treated mouse NK cell phenotype as compared to controls [83]. Taking into account the recently found relation between gut microbiota and Ps initiation, we have demonstrated that oral ingestion of IgY raised against pathological gut bacteria resistant to antibiotics can alleviate psoriatic lesions and restore immune parameters [18].

In Ps innate immune cells have been less studied in the peripheral circulation compared to lymphocytes. Besides KCs and T cells, neutrophils are an important cellular source of IL-17 via NETs formation in psoriatic lesions. NETs are increased in blood samples and were correlated with the severity of Ps [84]. Lambert et al. demonstrated that NETs promote Th17 cells induction from PBMCs in Ps. They also suggested that Th17 cells and neutrophils have a cross-talk because this effector helper subset produces cytokines that promote the development, recruitment, and lifespan of neutrophils [85].

Nguyen et al. observed a high expression of the co-stimulatory molecule CD86 on intermediate monocytes ($CD14^{++}CD16^{+}$) in Ps patients, along with high serum beta defensin-2 levels, these parameters positively correlated with PASI score [86]. Recent studies reported that low levels of monocytic myeloid-derived suppressor cells (Mo-MDSCs) are present in the peripheral blood of Ps patients; these cells secrete different pro-inflammatory cytokines (e.g. matrix metalloproteinases 9 and 1, IL-8) moderately suppressing $T\text{-}CD8^{+}$ cell proliferation. According to Soler et al., the immune system is unable to self-regulate due to the capability of Mo-MDSCs to induce aberrant Tregs cell conversion from naive T effector cells, in presence of pro-inflammatory molecules [87].

ILCs has a significantly increased frequency in the skin, but Villanova and al. observed in the blood of healthy individuals and Ps patients a large amount of CD3 negative ($CD3^{-}$) ILC who produce IL-17A and IL-22 (20% of IL-17 producing cells, respectively 40% of IL-22) [88]. $NKp44^{+}$ ILC3 group is the most frequent subset of ILCs in the peripheral blood and in the skin of Ps patients as compared to healthy individuals. The frequency of circulating NKp44+ ILC3 could reflect the disease severity and/or the response to anti-TNF treatment (adalimumab), highlighting the role of TNF in $NKp44^{+}$ ILC3 human differentiation [89].

Depending on the δ chain, γδT cells are classified into Vδ1–Vδ3 subsets. In the peripheral blood are present Vδ2 and Vδ3 groups, with the major subset Vγ9Vδ2 which produce a large range of pro-inflammatory mediators (e.g. IL-17A) and activate KCs in a TNF-α and IFN-γ dependent manner. Laggner et al. ha shown in peripheral blood a distinct subset of pro-inflammatory CLA and CCR6 positive Vγ9Vδ2 T cells, which are rapidly recruited into the injured skin [90]. These cells secrete IL-17 A,

IL-22 and activate KCs upon TNF-α, IFN-γ, and IL-23 stimulation [65]. Ps patients present low numbers of Vγ9Vδ2⁺ T cells in peripheral blood and concomitant high levels in psoriatic lesions, both suggesting the pathogenic role of the Vγ9Vδ2⁺ T subset [90]. The decreased concentration of circulating Vγ9Vδ2⁺ T cells is normalized after successful Ps treatment. All the data suggest a redistribution of these subsets of γδ T cells from blood to the skin [65].

3. Immune molecules as biomarkers in psoriasis

Ps is a polygenic skin disease with immunological etiology. The immune system interacts with KC and a complex network of cells is generated, where dendritic cells, T-lymphocytes, neutrophils, and mast cells communicate through immune-related molecules inducing the complex pathology of Ps. The main immune molecules involved in the development of this disease are IL-23, IL-17, IL-12, IL-22, IL-23, IL-6, IL-10, IFN, TNF, TGF-β1 [91]. All these molecules have cellular sources mainly Th17, Th22, and Tregs cells [92]. The presence of these molecules induces an inflammatory process that sustains the proliferation of epidermal cells, neo-angiogenesis, and infiltration of DCs in the skin. Recently, new players were identified in the Ps development, such as the skin microbiome [18] and the skin's serotonergic system [93]. For example, it was recently reported that the microbiome variations are associated with the level of inflammatory cytokines receptors, especially with the IL-2 receptor [94, 95].

A recent study has shown that Ps deregulated genes were found. These genes are involving cytokine-cytokine receptor interaction, cell cycle and cell adhesion molecules and these candidate genes regulating important immune pathways can be new therapeutic targets in Ps [96]. There are more than 50 genetic susceptible biomarkers associated with the risk of Ps. The strongest association is with the presence of the HLA-C*06 gene and HLA-B27 [97]. The other genetic Ps risk, single nucleotide polymorphisms (SNPs) are near the genes encoding molecules functioning in the adaptive and innate immunity [98].

3.1 Tissue immune molecules as biomarkers in psoriasis

The first cellular line of skin's defense is KCs that upon injury secrete an array of alarmins. These are molecules that induce a rapid innate immune response against danger signals. Any deregulation in the physiology of KCs can lead to chronic inflammation, hyper-proliferation, and eventually a psoriatic lesion. Keratins (KRTs), major structural intermediate filament proteins of KCs were shown to be involved in Ps. Hence, up-regulation of KRT6/16/17 induces hyper-proliferation and innate immune activation followed by autoimmune T cells activation [99]. Transcriptomic studies have shown that KCs from Ps skin harvested from patient's skin have a high expression of mRNA encoding for SERPINB [100]. Moreover, SERPINB is regulated by TEA domain family member 4 (TEAD4) and affects the secretion of chemokines in Ps, hindering the normal cross-talk between KCs and T cells [101]. Other important cells within the skin are dermal fibroblasts that are in close contact with immune cells. A recent proteomic study has shown that Ps fibroblasts have upregulated proinflammatory factors and downregulated other factors that are involved in transcription/translation processes, glycolysis/ adenosine triphosphate synthesis. All these deregulations contribute to the promotion of epidermal cell hyper-proliferation [102]. Another major cell involved in Ps is the Langerhans cell (LCs), the only DCs residing in the epidermis that is physically linked to KCs through E-cadherin. A recent study has shown that in Ps E-cadherin does not regulate LCs maturation, migration, and function [103].

There are a series of surface molecules appending to immune cells that are highly involved in Ps' appearance and maintenance of immune tolerance. Therefore, neuropilin-1 (NRP1), PD-1, and HLA-G are the main tissue players in Ps. These molecules were found significantly lower in Ps compared to normal skin and were similar in Ps variants like PsA and Ps vulgaris patients [104]. Another tissue immune marker relevant for Ps is the TLR superfamily. When TLRs become aberrantly activated, T cell-mediated autoimmune activation will take place, leading to several diseases including Ps [105]. In Ps' skin samples low levels of thrombospondin-1 (TSP-1) and CD47 were found inversely correlated with disease severity. The TSP-1/CD47 signaling pathway impacts Th17 and Tregs differentiation, favoring disease initiation [106]. Recently in an IMQ-induced psoriatic animal model, it was shown that IL-17A, IL-23, TNF-α, and STRA6 levels were found significantly increased in tissue along with their circulatory counterparts. RBP4 and STRA6 were found upregulated and involved in the experimental Ps [107]. The inflammatory Th17 response in Ps was reported to be modulated by IL-33 produced by the inflamed skin tissue, adding to the chronic status of Ps [108]. CDC6 is an essential regulator of the complex (pre-RC) assembly on chromatin. CDC6 expression was found upregulated in Ps lesions and probably the main route is induced by IL-22/STAT3 signaling, a key signaling pathway in Ps [109]. In a genetic mouse model, it was demonstrated that IL-23 produced by KCs induces chronic skin inflammation displaying an IL-17 pattern. In KCs from Ps' lesions, a decrease in H3K9 demethylation is correlated with IL-23 increased expression [110]. In a mouse experimental model harboring mutations in the gene encoding for CARD14 (KCs signaling molecule) it was shown that the animals spontaneously develop Ps, their skin has increased expression of anti-microbial peptides, chemokines, and cytokines, therefore Ps' pathogenesis in this model being driven by the IL-23/IL-17 axis. A diagram of the main immune molecules involved in Ps' pathogenesis is depicted in **Figure 3** [111].

In the IL-23/IL-17 axis, T lymphocytes, namely the Th17 subpopulation are the main cells that secrete IL-17A, IL-17F, and IL-22 [112], but also mast cells and neutrophils were shown to produce IL-17 in Ps' lesions [113].

3.2 Circulatory immune markers

Cytokines/chemokines that appear in the psoriatic lesion are essential for KCs activation. In immune homeostasis, if genetic and/or non-genetic factors interfere in the KC-T cell cross-talk the relation between resident T cells and KCs will be altered and a chronic inflammatory response will sustain the Ps lesions [114, 115]. All these alterations in terms of immune and non-immune molecules will be mirrored by the circulatory pattern of cytokines, chemokines, and various other molecules that can become biomarkers in Ps. A proteomic approach of Ps patients' plasma has shown that several proteins are decreased while others are increased. Hence apolipoprotein M, and proteins involved in vitamin D metabolism were found to decrease, while proteins involved in signaling molecule secretion were found to increase favoring cellular proliferation [116].

The complement system is essential in host defense against various pathogens, but in the last years, it was shown that due to its regulation properties of inflammation is involved in Ps development. As autoantibodies can activate the complement system, any deficiency of this system induces an impaired immune complex clearance and would sustain Ps lesions [117].

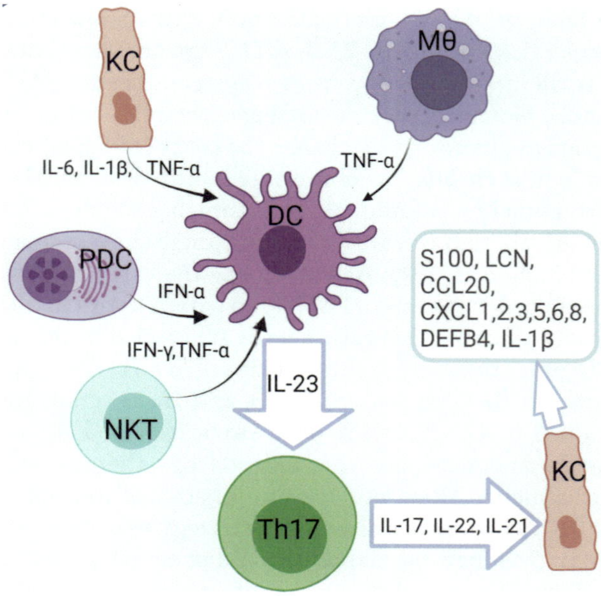

Figure 3.
IL-23/Th17 axis in Ps. DC are activated by various cells (KCs, Mϕ, PDC, NKT cells) and stimuli. When activated DC will secrete IL-23 activating Th17 lymphocytes that will activate KCs through IL-17, IL-22, IL-21. Activated KCs will express specific Ps' genes (DEFB4 gene which encoded human β-defensin 2) and secrete an array of molecules (S100 protein, lipocalin (LCN), CCL20, CXCL1-3, 5, 6, 8, IL-1β) that will induce chronic inflammation of the skin. Created with BioRender.com.

As already stated, the main deregulated axis in Ps is IL-22/IL-23/IL-17 axis. Memory Tregs are the main source of IL-17 in Ps [118]. IL-17A and F, when highly abundant, strongly induce S100-alarmins expression during KCs maturation [119]. IL-17A and IL-22 were found elevated in the serum of Ps patients, in accordance with increased IL-17 mRNA levels in the skin [120, 121]. IL-17A would further stimulate KCs to secrete chemokine CCL20, IL-8, and AMP, promoting inflammation [122]. Additionally, in Ps IL-17A synergizes with TNF and IL-22 and this cytokine cocktail upregulates IL-36 contributing to the inflammatory status [123]. IL-17F is found elevated in the serum of Ps [124] and is promoted by IL-23 [125], inducing further IL-6 and IL-8 secretion by KCs [126].

CD100-plexins were found elevated in Ps serum and were reported to increase the production of chemokines (CXCL1, CCL20) and cytokines (IL-1β, IL-18) when KCs activate NLRP3 inflammasome [127].

A recent study has shown that surviving, a protein belonging to the apoptosis inhibitor family was found to significantly increase in Ps patients suggesting its role in the pathogenesis of Ps [128].

4. Immune therapeutical outlines in Ps

Although diagnosis and therapy in skin pathologies have beneficiated from novel investigation assays [129, 130] and new therapies are emerging [18], there are still many immune niches that can be explored in the quest to find the best biomarker in diagnostic and therapy efficacy improvement [131].

A recent meta-analysis of biologics treatment in Ps has shown that the biological treatments that target IL-17, IL-12, IL-23, and TNF-α were significantly more effective in comparison to small molecules/conventional systemic agents [132]. Slowing down the pro-inflammatory biological processes using early intervention with anti-IL-17 and anti-IL-23 agents might positively change the course of Ps, especially in the current pandemic era, where chronic patients can reduce their hospital visits [133].

IL-17 inhibitors, namely secukinumab, ixekizumab, brodalumab and IL-23 inhibitors, namely guselkumab, tildrakizumab, risankizumab show increased effectiveness compared to other biologicals [134]. A recent meta-analysis has shown that these are the best choices in order to achieve PASI 90 in patients with moderate-to-severe psoriasis. The authors point out that future trials are needed to evaluate directly the biological agents in order to establish the best choice in terms of type and timing. Therefore, trials on anti-IL-17 versus anti-IL-23, anti-IL-23 versus anti-IL-12/-23, anti-TNF-α versus anti-IL-12/-23, and so on are to be expected (Cohrane skin group, 2021). Despite the therapeutical success of recent drugs, there are still a reactive patients to these treatments. Therefore, the combination of multiple immune-modulatory drugs can be an appropriate alternative strategy to improve the quality of life in Ps [135, 136]. Moreover, new biomarkers should personalize treatment with IL-17 inhibitors and IL-23 inhibitors and should stratify patients in Ps subgroups that could best beneficiate from these new biologics [137].

Historically, TNF-α inhibitors were the first biologicals approved in PsA. Now, targeting IL-12/IL-23 p40 common subunit, IL-17A, T cells co-stimulation, is proving an increased efficacy in Ps therapy. Moreover, additional drugs targeting phosphodiesterase-4 and JAK/STAT pathways are recently being developed [138]. Many cytokines are related to the pathways controlled by JAK/signal transducers and activators of transcription (STATs). JAK inhibitors have been approved in PsA [139]. In 2020, data from the Phase II trial of several selective TYK2 inhibitors in Ps were published [140] and new drugs targeting the JAK/STAT3 axis in Ps treatment are awaited [141]. Berberine was reported to inhibit CDK4/6-RB-CDC6 signaling in KCs, reducing their proliferation. This alkaloid extracted from Berberis plants represses JAK1, JAK2, and TYK2, inhibiting STAT3 activation [109].

Drug	Target	Stage	Reference
Anti-TNF	TNF-α	Approved	[132]
Secukinumab, ixekizumab, brodalumab	IL-17	Approved	[132, 133]
Guselkumab, tildrakizumab, risankizumab	IL-23		[134]
TYK2 inhibitors	TYK2	Phase II trial	[140]
Berberine	CDK4/6-RB-CDC6 signaling	In vitro experiments	[109]
Prostaglandin D2	Th2 cells	In vitro experiments	[144]
Luteolin	Proinflammatory cytokines	In vitro experiments	[146]

Table 1.
Main drugs approved in Ps and/or that are in various testing stages.

Co-stimulatory molecules (CD28, CD40, OX40, CD27, DR3, LFA-1, LFA-3) and co-inhibitory molecules (CTLA-4, PD-1, TIM-3) regulate T cells functions, including cytokines production and Tregs differentiation. In 2021 it was shown that co-signaling molecules targeting can be developed in future Ps' drugs [142].

Biologics targeting TNF, IL-17s, and IL-23 in Ps are associated with adverse immune effects. In a recent study, high antinuclear antibodies (ANA), high eosinophils, and high IgE were reported. Therefore, in Ps, careful observation is required when patients are subjected to these new biologics [143]. Due to these adverse effects, several other compounds are tested in Ps, like prostaglandin D2 inhibiting Th2 cells [144]. Vitamin D3 analogs, corticosteroids, or a combination of these compounds are tested as future drugs in Ps [145]. Flavonoids like luteolin can suppress proinflammatory cytokines (e.g., IL-1β, IL-6, IL-8, IL-17, IL-22, TNF-α) and regulate the signaling pathways that are highly involved in Ps [146].

Table 1 summarizes the main drugs that are already approved and/or are in various development stages in Ps.

5. Conclusion

Ps management is constantly evolving in parallel with new insights in the immune pathogenesis. In spite of extensive studies, Ps remains a complex and enigmatic disease as still, its clear etiology is a matter of intense research. New drugs that are targeting the immune pathways using biologics and small molecules have significantly improved life quality in Ps. Biomarkers from the area of cytokines, various soluble mediators, cell-surface molecules or receptors, intracellular signaling pathways molecules, encompass the panel of tools that can improve diagnosis and prognosis in Ps. The most recent image of Ps within the immunological system highlights the importance of immune cells involved in Ps.

Acknowledgements

This study was supported by the Core Program, implemented with the support of NASR, project PN 19.29.01.01 and 31PFE/31.12.2021.

Conflict of interest

The authors declare no conflict of interest.

Author details

Mihaela Surcel[1], Adriana Narcisa Munteanu[1,2], Carolina Constantin[1,3*] and Monica Neagu[1,2,3]

1 "Victor Babeș" National Institute of Pathology, Bucharest, Romania

2 Faculty of Biology, University of Bucharest, Romania

3 Colentina University Hospital, Bucharest, Romania

*Address all correspondence to: caroconstantin@gmail.com

References

[1] Parisi R, Symmons DPM, Griffiths CEM, Ashcroft DM. Global epidemiology of psoriasis: A systematic review of incidence and prevalence. The Journal of Investigative Dermatology. 2013;**133**(2):377-385

[2] Mehrmal S, Uppal P, Nedley N, Giesey RL, Delost GR. The global, regional, and national burden of psoriasis in 195 countries and territories, 1990 to 2017: A systematic analysis from the Global Burden of Disease Study 2017. Journal of the American Academy of Dermatology. 2021;**84**(1):46-52

[3] Tollefson MM, Crowson CS, McEvoy MT, Kremers HM. Incidence of psoriasis in children: A population-based study. Journal of the American Academy of Dermatology. 2010;**62**(6):1-17

[4] Ayala-Fontánez N, Soler DC, McCormick TS. Current knowledge on psoriasis and autoimmune diseases. Psoriasis (Auckl). 2016;**6**:7-32

[5] Kamiya K, Kishimoto M, Sugai J, Komine M, Ohtsuki M. Risk factors for the development of psoriasis. International Journal of Molecular Sciences. 2019;**20**(18):1-14

[6] Mylonas A, Conrad C. Psoriasis: Classical vs. paradoxical. The Yin-Yang of TNF and type I interferon. Frontiers in Immunology. 2018;**9**:1-10

[7] Lande R, Botti E, Jandus C, Dojcinovic D, Fanelli G, Conrad C, et al. The antimicrobial peptide LL37 is a T-cell autoantigen in psoriasis. Nature Communications. 2014;**5**:1-16

[8] Fuentes-Duculan J, Bonifacio KM, Hawkes JE, Kunjravia N, Cueto I, Li X, et al. Autoantigens ADAMTSL5 and LL37 are significantly upregulated in active psoriasis and localized with keratinocytes, dendritic cells and other leukocytes. Experimental Dermatology. 2017;**26**(11):1075-1082

[9] Jin L, Wang G. Keratin 17: A critical player in the pathogenesis of psoriasis. Medicinal Research Reviews. 2014;**34**(2):438-454

[10] Jablonska S, Chorzelski TP, Beutner EH, Maciejowska E, Jarzabek-Chorzelska null, Rzesa G. Autoimmunity in psoriasis. Relation of disease activity and forms of psoriasis to immunofluorescence findings. Archives of Dermatological Research. 1978;**261**(2):135-146

[11] Rambukkana A, Das PK, Witkamp L, Yong S, Meinardi MM, Bos JD. Antibodies to mycobacterial 65-kDa heat shock protein and other immunodominant antigens in patients with psoriasis. The Journal of Investigative Dermatology. 1993;**100**(1):87-92

[12] Di Meglio P, Villanova F, Nestle FO. Psoriasis. Cold Spring Harbor Perspectives in Medicine. 2014;**4**(8):1-30

[13] Korman NJ. Management of psoriasis as a systemic disease: What is the evidence? The British Journal of Dermatology. 2020;**182**(4):840-848

[14] Hawkes JE, Chan TC, Krueger JG. Psoriasis pathogenesis and the development of novel targeted immune therapies. The Journal of Allergy and Clinical Immunology. 2017;**140**(3):645-653

[15] Rendon A, Schäkel K. Psoriasis pathogenesis and treatment.

International Journal of Molecular Sciences. 2019;**20**(6):1-28

[16] Kovitwanichkanont T, Chong AH, Foley P. Beyond skin deep: Addressing comorbidities in psoriasis. The Medical Journal of Australia. 2020;**212**(11):528-534

[17] Osmancevic A, Ståhle M. Treatment of psoriasis: Before and now. Läkartidningen. 2017;**114**:EU6Y

[18] Surcel M, Munteanu A, Isvoranu G, Ibram A, Caruntu C, Constantin C, et al. Unconventional therapy with IgY in a psoriatic mouse model targeting gut microbiome. Journal of Personalized Medicine. 2021;**11**(9):1-21

[19] Morizane S, Gallo RL. Antimicrobial peptides in the pathogenesis of psoriasis. The Journal of Dermatology. 2012;**39**(3):225-230

[20] Chiang C-C, Cheng W-J, Korinek M, Lin C-Y, Hwang T-L. Neutrophils in psoriasis. Frontiers in Immunology. 2019;**10**:1-12

[21] Kennedy-Crispin M, Billick E, Mitsui H, Gulati N, Fujita H, Gilleaudeau P, et al. Human keratinocytes' response to injury upregulates CCL20 and other genes linking innate and adaptive immunity. The Journal of Investigative Dermatology. 2012;**132**(1):105-113

[22] Zaba LC, Fuentes-Duculan J, Eungdamrong NJ, Abello MV, Novitskaya I, Pierson KC, et al. Psoriasis is characterized by accumulation of immunostimulatory and Th1/Th17 cell polarizing myeloid dendritic cells. The Journal of Investigative Dermatology. 2009;**129**(1):79-88

[23] Mrowietz U. Neutrophils' sexiness is independent of trendy fashion. Experimental Dermatology. 2017;**26**(4):312-313

[24] Guo J, Tu J, Hu Y, Song G, Yin Z. Cathepsin G cleaves and activates IL-36γ and promotes the inflammation of psoriasis. Drug Design, Development and Therapy. 2019;**13**:581-588

[25] Dilek N, Dilek AR, Taşkın Y, Erkinüresin T, Yalçın Ö, Saral Y. Contribution of myeloperoxidase and inducible nitric oxide synthase to pathogenesis of psoriasis. Postępy Dermatologii i Alergologii. 2016;**33**(6): 435-439

[26] Lai R, Xian D, Xiong X, Yang L, Song J, Zhong J. Proanthocyanidins: Novel treatment for psoriasis that reduces oxidative stress and modulates Th17 and Treg cells. Redox Report. 2018;**23**(1):130-135

[27] Lin X, Huang T. Oxidative stress in psoriasis and potential therapeutic use of antioxidants. Free Radical Research. 2016;**50**(6):585-595

[28] Fuentes-Duculan J, Suárez-Fariñas M, Zaba LC, Nograles KE, Pierson KC, Mitsui H, et al. A subpopulation of CD163 positive macrophages is classically activated in psoriasis. The Journal of Investigative Dermatology. 2010;**130**(10):2412-2422

[29] Desplat-Jégo S, Burkly L, Putterman C. Targeting TNF and its family members in autoimmune/inflammatory disease. Mediators of Inflammation. 2014;**2014**:2. Article ID: 62874

[30] Ottaviani C, Nasorri F, Bedini C, de Pità O, Girolomoni G, Cavani A. CD56brightCD16(−) NK cells accumulate in psoriatic skin in response to CXCL10 and CCL5 and exacerbate skin inflammation. European Journal of Immunology. 2006;**36**(1):118-128

[31] Dunphy SE, Sweeney CM, Kelly G, Tobin AM, Kirby B, Gardiner CM. Natural killer cells from psoriasis vulgaris patients have reduced levels of cytotoxicity associated degranulation and cytokine production. Clinical Immunology. 2017;**177**:43-49

[32] Vissers WHPM, Berends M, Muys L, Van Erp PEJ, De Jong EMGJ, Van De Kerkhof PCM. The effect of the combination of calcipotriol and betamethasone dipropionate versus both monotherapies on epidermal proliferation, keratinization and T-cell subsets in chronic plaque psoriasis. Experimental Dermatology. 2004;**13**(2):106-112

[33] Bonish B, Jullien D, Dutronc Y, Huang BB, Modlin R, Spada FM, et al. Overexpression of CD1d by keratinocytes in psoriasis and CD1d-dependent IFN-gamma production by NK-T cells. Journal of Immunology. 2000;**165**(7):4076-4085

[34] Tsagaratou A. Unveiling the regulation of NKT17 cell differentiation and function. Molecular Immunology. 2019;(105):55-61

[35] Vivier E, Artis D, Colonna M, Diefenbach A, Di Santo JP, Eberl G, et al. Innate lymphoid cells: 10 years on. Cell. 2018;**174**(5):1054-1066

[36] Villanova F, Flutter B, Tosi I, Grys K, Sreeneebus H, Perera GK, et al. Characterization of innate lymphoid cells in human skin and blood demonstrates increase of NKp44+ ILC3 in psoriasis. The Journal of Investigative Dermatology. 2014;**134**(4):984-991

[37] Teunissen MBM, Munneke JM, Bernink JH, Spuls PI, Res PCM, Te Velde A, et al. Composition of innate lymphoid cell subsets in the human skin: Enrichment of NCR(+) ILC3 in lesional skin and blood of psoriasis patients. The Journal of Investigative Dermatology. 2014;**134**(9):2351-2360

[38] Bonneville M, O'Brien RL, Born WK. γδ T cell effector functions: A blend of innate programming and acquired plasticity. Nature Reviews. Immunology. 2010;**10**(7):467-478

[39] Papotto PH, Reinhardt A, Prinz I, Silva-Santos B. Innately versatile: γδ17 T cells in inflammatory and autoimmune diseases. Journal of Autoimmunity. 2018;**87**:26-37

[40] Cai Y, Shen X, Ding C, Qi C, Li K, Li X, et al. Pivotal role of dermal IL-17-producing γδ T cells in skin inflammation. Immunity. 2011;**35**(4):596-610

[41] Matos TR, O'Malley JT, Lowry EL, Hamm D, Kirsch IR, Robins HS, et al. Clinically resolved psoriatic lesions contain psoriasis-specific IL-17–producing αβ T cell clones. Journal of Clinical Investigation;**127**(11):4031-4041

[42] Grän F, Kerstan A, Serfling E, Goebeler M, Muhammad K. Current developments in the immunology of psoriasis. The Yale Journal of Biology and Medicine. 2020;**93**(1):97-110

[43] Casciano F, Pigatto PD, Secchiero P, Gambari R, Reali E. T cell hierarchy in the pathogenesis of psoriasis and associated cardiovascular comorbidities. Frontiers in Immunology. 2018;**9**:1390-1398

[44] Valdimarsson H, Thorleifsdottir RH, Sigurdardottir SL, Gudjonsson JE, Johnston A. Psoriasis—As an autoimmune disease caused by molecular mimicry. Trends in Immunology. 2009;**30**(10):494-501

[45] Gallais Sérézal I, Classon C, Cheuk S, Barrientos-Somarribas M,

Wadman E, Martini E, et al. Resident T cells in resolved psoriasis steer tissue responses that stratify clinical outcome. Journal of Investigative Dermatology. 2018;**138**(8):1754-1763

[46] Di Meglio P, Villanova F, Navarini AA, Mylonas A, Tosi I, Nestle FO, et al. Targeting CD8+ T cells prevents psoriasis development. The Journal of Allergy and Clinical Immunology. 2016;**138**(1):1-9

[47] Schlaak JF, Buslau M, Jochum W, Hermann E, Girndt M, Gallati H, et al. T cells involved in psoriasis vulgaris belong to the Th1 subset. The Journal of Investigative Dermatology. 1994;**102**(2):145-149

[48] Kryczek I, Bruce AT, Gudjonsson JE, Johnston A, Aphale A, Vatan L, et al. Induction of IL-17+ T cell trafficking and development by IFN-γ: Mechanism and pathological relevance in psoriasis. Journal of Immunology. 2008;**181**(7):4733-4741

[49] Chung Y, Chang SH, Martinez GJ, Yang XO, Nurieva R, Kang HS, et al. Critical regulation of early Th17 cell differentiation by interleukin-1 signaling. Immunity. 2009;**30**(4):576-587

[50] Harden JL, Johnson-Huang LM, Chamian MF, Lee E, Pearce T, Leonardi CL, et al. Humanized anti–IFN-γ (HuZAF) in the treatment of psoriasis. The Journal of Allergy and Clinical Immunology. 2015;**135**(2):553-556

[51] Li B, Huang L, Lv P, Li X, Liu G, Chen Y, et al. The role of Th17 cells in psoriasis. Immunologic Research. 2020;**68**(5):296-309

[52] Boutet M-A, Nerviani A, Gallo Afflitto G, Pitzalis C. Role of the IL-23/IL-17 Axis in psoriasis and psoriatic arthritis: The clinical importance of its divergence in skin and joints. International Journal of Molecular Sciences. 2018;**19**(2):530-557

[53] Bettelli E, Oukka M, Kuchroo VK. T(H)-17 cells in the circle of immunity and autoimmunity. Nature Immunology. 2007;**8**(4):345-350

[54] Lowes MA, Kikuchi T, Fuentes-Duculan J, Cardinale I, Zaba LC, Haider AS, et al. Psoriasis vulgaris lesions contain discrete populations of Th1 and Th17 T cells. The Journal of Investigative Dermatology. 2008;**128**(5):1207-1211

[55] Yawalkar N, Tscharner GG, Hunger RE, Hassan AS. Increased expression of IL-12p70 and IL-23 by multiple dendritic cell and macrophage subsets in plaque psoriasis. Journal of Dermatological Science. 2009;**54**(2):99-105

[56] Lowes MA, Suárez-Fariñas M, Krueger JG. Immunology of psoriasis. Annual Review of Immunology. 2014;**32**:227-255

[57] Cheuk S, Wikén M, Blomqvist L, Nylén S, Talme T, Ståhle M, et al. Epidermal Th22 and Tc17 cells form a localized disease memory in clinically healed psoriasis. Journal of Immunology. 2014;**192**(7):3111-3120

[58] Cai Y, Fleming C, Yan J. New insights of T cells in the pathogenesis of psoriasis. Cellular & Molecular Immunology. 2012;**9**(4):302-309

[59] Nussbaum L, Chen Y, Ogg G. Role of regulatory T cells in psoriasis pathogenesis and treatment. The British Journal of Dermatology. 2021;**184**(1):14-24

[60] Bovenschen HJ, van de Kerkhof PC, van Erp PE, Woestenenk R, Joosten I,

Koenen HJPM. Foxp3+ regulatory T cells of psoriasis patients easily differentiate into IL-17A-producing cells and are found in lesional skin. The Journal of Investigative Dermatology. 2011;**131**(9):1853-1860

[61] Gray D, Gray M. What are regulatory B cells? European Journal of Immunology. 2010;**40**(10):2677-2679

[62] Yanaba K, Kamata M, Ishiura N, Shibata S, Asano Y, Tada Y, et al. Regulatory B cells suppress imiquimod-induced, psoriasis-like skin inflammation. Journal of Leukocyte Biology. 2013;**94**(4):563-573

[63] Priyadarssini M, Divya Priya D, Indhumathi S, Rajappa M, Chandrashekar L, Thappa DM. Immunophenotyping of T cells in the peripheral circulation in psoriasis. British Journal of Biomedical Science. 2016;**73**(4):174-179

[64] Zhu K, Ye J, Wu M, Cheng H. Expression of Th1 and Th2 cytokine-associated transcription factors, T-bet and GATA-3, in peripheral blood mononuclear cells and skin lesions of patients with psoriasis vulgaris. Archives of Dermatological Research. 2010;**302**(7):517-523

[65] Das D, Akhtar S, Kurra S, Gupta S, Sharma A. Emerging role of immune cell network in autoimmune skin disorders: An update on pemphigus, vitiligo and psoriasis. Cytokine & Growth Factor Reviews. 2019;**45**:35-44

[66] Wang Y, Wang L-L, Yang H-Y, Wang F-F, Zhang X-X, Bai Y-P. Interleukin-21 is associated with the severity of psoriasis vulgaris through promoting CD4+ T cells to differentiate into Th17 cells. American Journal of Translational Research. 2016;**8**(7):3188-3196

[67] Luan L, Ding Y, Han S, Zhang Z, Liu X. An increased proportion of circulating Th22 and Tc22 cells in psoriasis. Cellular Immunology. 2014;**290**(2):196-200

[68] Karamehic J, Zecevic L, Resic H, Jukic M, Jukic T, Ridjic O, et al. Immunophenotype lymphocyte of peripheral blood in patients with psoriasis. Medical Archives. 2014;**68**(4):236-238

[69] Zhang L, Yang X-Q, Cheng J, Hui R-S, Gao T-W. Increased Th17 cells are accompanied by FoxP3+ Treg cell accumulation and correlated with psoriasis disease severity. Clinical Immunology. 2010;**135**(1):108-117

[70] Yun W-J, Lee D-W, Chang S-E, Yoon G-S, Huh J-R, Won C-H, et al. Role of CD4CD25FOXP3 regulatory T cells in psoriasis. Annals of Dermatology. 2010;**22**(4):397-403

[71] Crotty S. T follicular helper cell differentiation, function, and roles in disease. Immunity. 2014;**41**(4):529-542

[72] Shin D, Kim DS, Kim SH, Je JH, Kim HJ, Young Kim D, et al. Decreased PD-1 positive blood follicular helper T cells in patients with psoriasis. Archives of Dermatological Research. 2016;**308**(8):593-599

[73] Sigmundsdóttir H, Gudjónsson JE, Jónsdóttir I, Lúdvíksson BR, Valdimarsson H. The frequency of CLA+ CD8+ T cells in the blood of psoriasis patients correlates closely with the severity of their disease. Clinical and Experimental Immunology. 2001;**126**(2):365-369

[74] Colombo E, Galleri G, Erre GL, Piras C, Biondi G, Taras L, et al. Peripheral blood CD8+ T-cell profiles in patients with psoriatic arthritis:

A cross-sectional case-control study. European Review for Medical and Pharmacological Sciences. 2017;**21**(22): 5166-5171

[75] Lu J, Ding Y, Yi X, Zheng J. CD19+ B cell subsets in the peripheral blood and skin lesions of psoriasis patients and their correlations with disease severity. Brazilian Journal of Medical and Biological Research. 2016;**49**(9):1-9

[76] Mavropoulos A, Varna A, Zafiriou E, Liaskos C, Alexiou I, Roussaki-Schulze A, et al. IL-10 producing Bregs are impaired in psoriatic arthritis and psoriasis and inversely correlate with IL-17- and IFNγ-producing T cells. Clinical Immunology. 2017;**184**:33-41

[77] Mavropoulos A, Zafiriou E, Simopoulou T, Brotis AG, Liaskos C, Roussaki-Schulze A, et al. Apremilast increases IL-10-producing regulatory B cells and decreases proinflammatory T cells and innate cells in psoriatic arthritis and psoriasis. Rheumatology (Oxford, England). 2019;**58**(12):2240-2250

[78] Sato Y, Ogawa E, Okuyama R. Role of innate immune cells in psoriasis. International Journal of Molecular Sciences. 2020;**21**(18):1-17

[79] Dunphy S, Gardiner CM. NK cells and psoriasis. Journal of Biomedicine & Biotechnology. 2011;**2011**:1-10

[80] Skrzeczyńska-Moncznik J, Stefańska A, Zabel BA, Kapińska-Mrowiecka M, Butcher EC, Cichy J. Chemerin and the recruitment of NK cells to diseased skin. Acta Biochimica Polonica. 2009;**56**(2):355-360

[81] Gambichler T, Zhang Y, Höxtermann S, Kreuter A. Natural killer cells and B lymphocytes in peripheral blood of patients with psoriasis. The British Journal of Dermatology. 2013;**168**(4):894-896

[82] Surcel M, Huică R-I, Munteanu AN, Isvoranu G, Pîrvu IR, Ciotaru D, et al. Phenotypic changes of lymphocyte populations in psoriasiform dermatitis animal model. Experimental and Therapeutic Medicine. 2019;**17**(2): 1030-1038

[83] Surcel M, Munteanu AN, Huică R-I, Isvoranu G, Pîrvu IR, Constantin C, et al. Reinforcing involvement of NK cells in psoriasiform dermatitis animal model. Experimental and Therapeutic Medicine. 2019;**18**(6):4956-4966

[84] Lee KH, Kronbichler A, Park DD-Y, Park Y, Moon H, Kim H, et al. Neutrophil extracellular traps (NETs) in autoimmune diseases: A comprehensive review. Autoimmunity Reviews. 2017;**16**(11):1160-1173

[85] Lambert S, Hambro CA, Johnston A, Stuart PE, Tsoi LC, Nair RP, et al. Neutrophil extracellular traps induce human Th17 cells: Effect of psoriasis-associated TRAF3IP2 genotype. Journal of Investigative Dermatology. 2019;**139**(6):1245-1253

[86] Nguyen CTH, Kambe N, Yamazaki F, Ueda-Hayakawa I, Kishimoto I, Okamoto H. Up-regulated expression of CD86 on circulating intermediate monocytes correlated with disease severity in psoriasis. Journal of Dermatological Science. 2018;**90**(2):135-143

[87] Soler DC, Young AB, Fiessinger L, Galimberti F, Debanne S, Groft S, et al. Increased, but functionally impaired, CD14+ HLA-DR−/low myeloid-derived suppressor cells in psoriasis: A mechanism of dysregulated T cells. Journal of Investigative Dermatology. 2016;**136**(4):798-808

[88] Villanova F, Flutter B, Tosi I, Grys K, Sreeneebus H, Perera GK, et al. Characterization of innate lymphoid cells (ILC) in human skin and blood demonstrates increase of NKp44+ ILC3 in psoriasis. The Journal of Investigative Dermatology. 2014;**134**(4):984-991

[89] Bernink JH, Peters CP, Munneke M, te Velde AA, Meijer SL, Weijer K, et al. Human type 1 innate lymphoid cells accumulate in inflamed mucosal tissues. Nature Immunology. 2013;**14**(3):221-229

[90] Laggner U, Di Meglio P, Perera GK, Hundhausen C, Lacy KE, Ali N, et al. Identification of a novel proinflammatory human skin-homing Vγ9Vδ2 T cell subset with a potential role in psoriasis. Journal of Immunology. 2011;**187**(5):2783-2793

[91] Surcel M, Huica R, Constantin C, Neagu CU. Biomarkers insights in psoriasis—regulatory cytokines. Current Biomarkers. 2017;**7**(1):1-9

[92] Georgescu S-R, Tampa M, Caruntu C, Sarbu M-I, Mitran C-I, Mitran M-I, et al. Advances in understanding the immunological pathways in psoriasis. International Journal of Molecular Sciences. 2019;**20**(3):1-17

[93] Martins AM, Ascenso A, Ribeiro HM, Marto J. The brain–skin connection and the pathogenesis of psoriasis: A review with a focus on the serotonergic system. Cell. 2020;**9**(4):1-23

[94] Mann EA, Bae E, Kostyuchek D, Chung HJ, McGee JS. The gut microbiome: Human health and inflammatory skin diseases. Annals of Dermatology. 2020;**32**(4):265-272

[95] Zhang X, Shi L, Sun T, Guo K, Geng S. Dysbiosis of gut microbiota and its correlation with dysregulation of cytokines in psoriasis patients. BMC Microbiology. 2021;**21**(1):1-10

[96] Choudhary S, Anand R, Pradhan D, Bastia B, Kumar SN, Singh H, et al. Transcriptomic landscaping of core genes and pathways of mild and severe psoriasis vulgaris. International Journal of Molecular Medicine. 2021;**47**(1):219-231

[97] Caso F, Costa L, Chimenti MS, Navarini L, Punzi L. Pathogenesis of psoriatic arthritis. CRI. 2019;**39**(5): 361-377

[98] Nedoszytko B, Szczerkowska-Dobosz A, Stawczyk-Macieja M, Owczarczyk-Saczonek A, Reich A, Bartosińska J, et al. Pathogenesis of psoriasis in the 'omic' era. Part II. Genetic, genomic and epigenetic changes in psoriasis. Postępy Dermatologii i Alergologii. 2020;**37**(3):283-298

[99] Zhang X, Yin M, Zhang L. Keratin 6, 16 and 17—Critical barrier Alarmin molecules in skin wounds and psoriasis. Cell. 2019;**8**(8):1-14

[100] Wang Z, Zheng H, Zhou H, Huang N, Wei X, Liu X, et al. Systematic screening and identification of novel psoriasis-specific genes from the transcriptome of psoriasis-like keratinocytes. Molecular Medicine Reports. 2019;**19**(3):1529-1542

[101] Ren C, Liu Q, Ma Y, Wang A, Yang Y, Wang D. TEAD4 transcriptional regulates SERPINB3/4 and affect crosstalk between keratinocytes and T cells in psoriasis. Immunobiology. 2020;**225**(5):1-8

[102] Gęgotek A, Domingues P, Wroński A, Skrzydlewska E. Changes in proteome of fibroblasts isolated from psoriatic skin lesions. International Journal of Molecular Sciences. 2020; **21**(15):1-17

[103] Brand A, Diener N, Zahner SP, Tripp C, Backer RA, Karram K, et al. E-cadherin is dispensable to maintain Langerhans cells in the epidermis. The Journal of Investigative Dermatology. 2020;**140**(1):132-142

[104] Bartosińska J, Purkot J, Kowal M, Michalak-Stoma A, Krasowska D, Chodorowska G, et al. The expression of selected molecular markers of immune tolerance in psoriatic patients. Advances in Clinical and Experimental Medicine. 2018;**27**(6):721-725

[105] Sun L, Liu W, Zhang L. The role of toll-like receptors in skin host defense, psoriasis, and atopic dermatitis. Journal of Immunology Research. 2019;**2019**:1-14

[106] Rodríguez-Jiménez P, Chicharro P, Llamas-Velasco M, Cibrian D, Trigo-Torres L, Vara A, et al. Thrombospondin-1/CD47 interaction regulates Th17 and Treg differentiation in psoriasis. Frontiers in Immunology. 2019;**10**:1-10

[107] Wang H, Wu C, Jiang Y, Wang W, Jin H. Retinol and vitamin a metabolites accumulate through RBP4 and STRA6 changes in a psoriasis murine model. Nutrition and Metabolism. 2020;**17**(1):1-15

[108] Milling S, Siebert S. T cells and cytokines in inflamed psoriatic skin. Who's in charge? Immunology. 2020;**160**(4):311-312

[109] Sun S, Zhang X, Xu M, Zhang F, Tian F, Cui J, et al. Berberine downregulates CDC6 and inhibits proliferation via targeting JAK-STAT3 signaling in keratinocytes. Cell Death & Disease. 2019;**10**(4):1-16

[110] Li H, Yao Q, Mariscal AG, Wu X, Hülse J, Pedersen E, et al. Epigenetic control of IL-23 expression in keratinocytes is important for chronic skin inflammation. Nature Communications. 2018;**9**(1):1-18

[111] Mellett M, Meier B, Mohanan D, Schairer R, Cheng P, Satoh TK, et al. CARD14 gain-of-function mutation alone is sufficient to drive IL-23/IL-17-mediated Psoriasiform skin inflammation In vivo. The Journal of Investigative Dermatology. 2018;**138**(9):2010-2023

[112] Boehncke W-H, Schön MP. Psoriasis. The Lancet. 2015;**386**(9997):983-994

[113] Lin AM, Rubin CJ, Khandpur R, Wang JY, Riblett M, Yalavarthi S, et al. Mast cells and neutrophils release IL-17 through extracellular trap formation in psoriasis. Journal of Immunology. 2011;**187**(1):490-500

[114] Albanesi C, Madonna S, Gisondi P, Girolomoni G. The interplay between keratinocytes and immune cells in the pathogenesis of psoriasis. Frontiers in Immunology. 2018;**9**:1-7

[115] Caruntu C, Boda D, Dumitrascu G, Constantin C, Neagu M. Proteomics focusing on immune markers in psoriatic arthritis. Biomarkers in Medicine. 2014;**9**(6):513-528

[116] Gęgotek A, Domingues P, Wroński A, Wójcik P, Skrzydlewska E. Proteomic plasma profile of psoriatic patients. Journal of Pharmaceutical and Biomedical Analysis. 2018;**155**:185-193

[117] Giang J, Seelen MAJ, van Doorn MBA, Rissmann R, Prens EP, Damman J. Complement activation in inflammatory skin diseases. Frontiers in Immunology. 2018;**9**:1-17

[118] Esmaeili B, Mansouri P, Meysamie A, Izad M. Evaluation of IL-17 producing memory regulatory and

effector T cells expressing CD26 molecule in patients with psoriasis. Iranian Journal of Allergy, Asthma, and Immunology. 2018;**17**:453-463

[119] Christmann C, Zenker S, Martens L, Hübner J, Loser K, Vogl T, et al. Interleukin 17 promotes expression of Alarmins S100A8 and S100A9 during the inflammatory response of keratinocytes. Frontiers in Immunology. 2021;**11**:1-16

[120] Li J, Li D, Tan Z. The expression of interleukin-17, interferon-gamma, and macrophage inflammatory protein-3 alpha mRNA in patients with psoriasis vulgaris. Journal of Huazhong University of Science and Technology. Medical Sciences. 2004;**24**(3):294-296

[121] Johansen C, Usher PA, Kjellerup RB, Lundsgaard D, Iversen L, Kragballe K. Characterization of the interleukin-17 isoforms and receptors in lesional psoriatic skin. The British Journal of Dermatology. 2009;**160**(2):319-324

[122] Ivanov S, Lindén A. Interleukin-17 as a drug target in human disease. Trends in Pharmacological Sciences. 2009;**30**(2):95-103

[123] Chiricozzi A, Guttman-Yassky E, Suárez-Fariñas M, Nograles KE, Tian S, Cardinale I, et al. Integrative responses to IL-17 and TNF-α in human keratinocytes account for key inflammatory pathogenic circuits in psoriasis. The Journal of Investigative Dermatology. 2011;**131**(3):677-687

[124] Soderstrom C, Berstein G, Zhang W, Valdez H, Fitz L, Kuhn M, et al. Ultra-sensitive measurement of IL-17A and IL-17F in psoriasis patient serum and skin. The AAPS Journal. 2017;**19**(4):1218-1222

[125] Aggarwal S, Ghilardi N, Xie M-H, de Sauvage FJ, Gurney AL. Interleukin-23 promotes a distinct CD4 T cell activation state characterized by the production of interleukin-17. The Journal of Biological Chemistry. 2003;**278**(3):1910-1914

[126] Fujishima S, Watanabe H, Kawaguchi M, Suzuki T, Matsukura S, Homma T, et al. Involvement of IL-17F via the induction of IL-6 in psoriasis. Archives of Dermatological Research. 2010;**302**(7):499-505

[127] Zhang C, Xiao C, Dang E, Cao J, Zhu Z, Fu M, et al. CD100-Plexin-B2 promotes the inflammation in psoriasis by activating NF-κB and the inflammasome in keratinocytes. The Journal of Investigative Dermatology. 2018;**138**(2):375-383

[128] Akpinar U, Gur Aksoy G, Hayran Y, Firat Oguz E, Yalcın B. Serum levels of survivin in patients with psoriasis and their relation to disease characteristics. Journal of Cosmetic Dermatology. 2021:1-6

[129] Ilie MA, Caruntu C, Lupu M, Lixandru D, Tampa M, Georgescu S-R, et al. Current and future applications of confocal laser scanning microscopy imaging in skin oncology. Oncology Letters. 2019;**17**(5):4102-4211

[130] Ghita MA, Caruntu C, Rosca AE, Kaleshi H, Caruntu A, Moraru L, et al. Reflectance confocal microscopy and dermoscopy for in vivo, non-invasive skin imaging of superficial basal cell carcinoma. Oncology Letters. 2016;**11**(5):3019-3024

[131] Neagu M. The immune system--a hidden treasure for biomarker discovery in cutaneous melanoma. Advances in Clinical Chemistry. 2012;**58**:89-140

[132] Sbidian E, Chaimani A, Afach S, Doney L, Dressler C, Hua C, et al. Systemic pharmacological treatments for chronic plaque psoriasis: A network

meta-analysis. Cochrane Database of Systematic Reviews. 2020;**1**:1-602

[133] Magina S, Filipe P. Pathophysiology of moderate to severe plaque psoriasis: Anti-IL-17 towards disease modification. Drugs Today. 2021;**57**(5):347-357

[134] Radi G, Campanati A, Diotallevi F, Bianchelli T, Offidani A. Novel therapeutic approaches and targets for treatment of psoriasis. Current Pharmaceutical Biotechnology. 2021;**22**(1):7-31

[135] Pastor-Fernández G, Mariblanca IR, Navarro MN. Decoding IL-23 signaling cascade for new therapeutic opportunities. Cell. 2020;**9**(9):1-33

[136] Iznardo H, Puig L. Dual inhibition of IL-17A and IL-17F in psoriatic disease. Therapeutic Advances in Chronic Disease. 2021;**12**:1-16

[137] Gisondi P, Geat D, Pizzolato M, Girolomoni G. State of the art and pharmacological pipeline of biologics for chronic plaque psoriasis. Current Opinion in Pharmacology. 2019;**46**:90-99

[138] Silvagni E, Bortoluzzi A, Ciancio G, Govoni M. Biological and synthetic target DMARDs in psoriatic arthritis. Pharmacological Research. 2019;**149**:1-46

[139] Fragoulis GE, McInnes IB, Siebert S, JAK-inhibitors. New players in the field of immune-mediated diseases, beyond rheumatoid arthritis. Rheumatology (Oxford, England). 2019;**58**(Suppl. 1): 43-54

[140] Nogueira M, Puig L, Torres T. JAK inhibitors for treatment of psoriasis: Focus on selective TYK2 inhibitors. Drugs. 2020;**80**(4):341-352

[141] Calautti E, Avalle L, Poli V. Psoriasis: A STAT3-centric view. International Journal of Molecular Sciences. 2018;**19**(1):1-14

[142] Liu S, Xu J, Wu J. The role of co-signaling molecules in psoriasis and their implications for targeted treatment. Frontiers in Pharmacology. 2021;**12**:1-11

[143] Sugiura R, Terui H, Shimada-Omori R, Yamazaki E, Tsuchiyama K, Takahashi T, et al. Biologics modulate antinuclear antibodies, immunoglobulin E, and eosinophil counts in psoriasis patients. The Journal of Dermatology. 2021;**48**(11):1739-1744

[144] Honda T, Kabashima K. Prostanoids and leukotrienes in the pathophysiology of atopic dermatitis and psoriasis. International Immunology. 2019;**31**(9):589-595

[145] Singh A, Easwari TS. Recent advances in psoriasis therapy: Trends and future prospects. Current Drug Targets. 2021;**22**(15):1760-1771

[146] Gendrisch F, Esser PR, Schempp CM, Wölfle U. Luteolin as a modulator of skin aging and inflammation. BioFactors. 2021;**47**(2):170-180

Chapter 6

Immunomodulatory Effect of Methotrexate Abruptly Controls Keratinocyte Activation in Psoriasis

Tamilselvi Elango, Anburaj Jeyaraj, Haripriya Dayalan, Pushpa Gnanaraj, Xinghui Li and Xuejun Zhang

Abstract

In psoriatic skin, epidermal keratinocytes (KCs) undergo deregulated inflammatory response that leads to prolonged expression of inflammatory mediators as well as abnormal keratins. Due to immune and genetic factors, KCs get activated and cell balance gets disturbed. This activation is mainly due to deregulated inflammatory response. A vicious cycle of KC-immune response called KC activation cycle leads to psoriasis. In psoriatic skin, epidermal KCs undergo deregulated inflammatory response that leads to prolonged expression of inflammatory mediators as well as abnormal keratins. Methotrexate (MTX) an immunosuppressive agent has been used as a standard drug to treat severe psoriasis. Acanthosis and abnormal terminal differentiation was mainly due to the mutation in epidermal keratins. In turn, disease severity and relapsing of psoriasis are mainly due to the mutation of hyperproliferative keratins. These novel keratin mutations in psoriatic epidermis might be one of the causative factors for psoriasis. MTX strongly regulates the KC activation cycle by deregulated inflammatory markers and maintains normal keratin phenotype on hyperproliferating KC, thereby controlling acanthosis in psoriasis patients.

Keywords: psoriasis, methotrexate, keratins, inflammatory markers, keratinocyte

1. Introduction

Psoriasis is a chronic inflammatory skin disease that mainly characterized by acanthosis, abnormal differentiation and infiltration of leukocytes from the dermis. The factors that causing this disease are genetic, environmental and inflammatory mediators [1]. In normal skin, the transformation of basal keratinocytes (KCs) to anucleate corneocytes process will takes within 50 days. Whereas, in psoriatic skin the epidermal cell cycle is rapid and the transformation occurs within 5 days. Thereby, the stratum corneum contains fully unmatured keratinized cells which build up abnormally and forms scales like structure. Due to this, epidermis of psoriatic lesions will become thicker and also blood vessels in the papillary layer of the dermis get dilated along with effusion of inflammatory cells, such as neutrophils, infiltrate the epidermis [2]. About 80% of the epidermal skin constitutes KCs. KC play a major role in this chronic inflammatory disease. It play a special role in sensing epidermal barrier and regulating immune homeostasis [1].

1.1 Hyperproliferation of epidermis in psoriasis

Until the late 1970s, the hypothesis of psoriasis arising from abnormalities in KCs was favored, and the abnormal proliferation was treated with antiproliferative agents. Since then, the participation of KC in the pathogenesis of psoriasis has certainly been overlooked. A publication by Zenz et al. [3] has highlighted again the role of KC in the pathomechanisms leading to psoriatic lesions. Their findings favor the view that psoriasis could also be regarded as a primary KC disorder amplified by the immune system [4]. While the debate will continue among skin biologists on the different theories, it is unquestionable that KC are potential initiators of inflammation, producing a number of cytokines, adhesion molecules and growth factors.

The growth of KC is regulated by a delicate balance between molecules that control cell survival and cell death. Thus, the thickness of human epidermis remains relatively constant throughout life. This regulation is disturbed in psoriasis that leads to KC hyperproliferation with the net result of an increase in the volume of cell mass [5]. The epidermal cell cycle of hyperproliferating psoriatic KC occurs within 5 days. Effusion of growth factors and inflammatory mediators from different skin cells, are believed to regulate the epidermal hyperproliferation in psoriasis (**Figure 1**) [6].

When skin cells exposed to any external factors such as environmental, chemical and internal factor like genetic, psychological and physical stress will probably activate immune cells within the KCs, which create KCs to hyperproliferate and also altered differentiation. Thus, the establishment of mutual KC-immunocyte stimulation (KC activation cycle) will leads to psoriasis [7, 8]. The hyperproliferation in psoriasis seemed to result from an increase in the number of transit amplifying cells, following depletion of the stem cell compartment [9]. As a whole, these changes suggest that intermediate filament (IF) keratin pair provides specific functional requirements to maintain epidermal KCs. KCs stability and integrity are mainly depend on keratin proteins [10, 11]. Keratins are the main structural cytoskeletal protein, an IF in all epithelia [12]. In normal skin, basal KCs express K5 and Keratin 14 (K14) keratins which helps in proliferation, whereas suprabasal cells express K1 and Keratin 10 (K10) keratins which supports differentiation process [13, 14]. Subsequently, any defects in these keratins can lead to cell fragility and are linked to a wide array of genodermatoses and cancers [15, 16].

Since genome-wide association studies (GWAS), connecting the psoriasis to the late cornified envelope gene cluster has specified that epidermal abnormalities along with hyperproliferative keratin pattern plays a major role in the pathogenesis of psoriasis [17, 18]. Studies have shown that dysfunction or mutations of keratin proteins are associated with a remarkable variety of skin disorders, such as skin blistering, inflammatory disorders and skin tumors [19]. The main aim of psoriasis treatments is to stop skin cells from growing so quickly and to remove scales. Methotrexate (MTX) is considered as the gold standard therapy for moderate to severe psoriasis [20–23]. Mostly, MTX exerts various immunomodulatory effects on T cell and also control KC growth [24]. In psoriasis, MTX was found to decreases the markers involved in hyperproliferation [25].

In this chapter we will first describe KC hyperproliferation then how keratins are expressed and regulated in psoriasis, then we will describe how MTX exert its action on controlling psoriasis through its immunomodulatory effect on Keratins and KC activation.

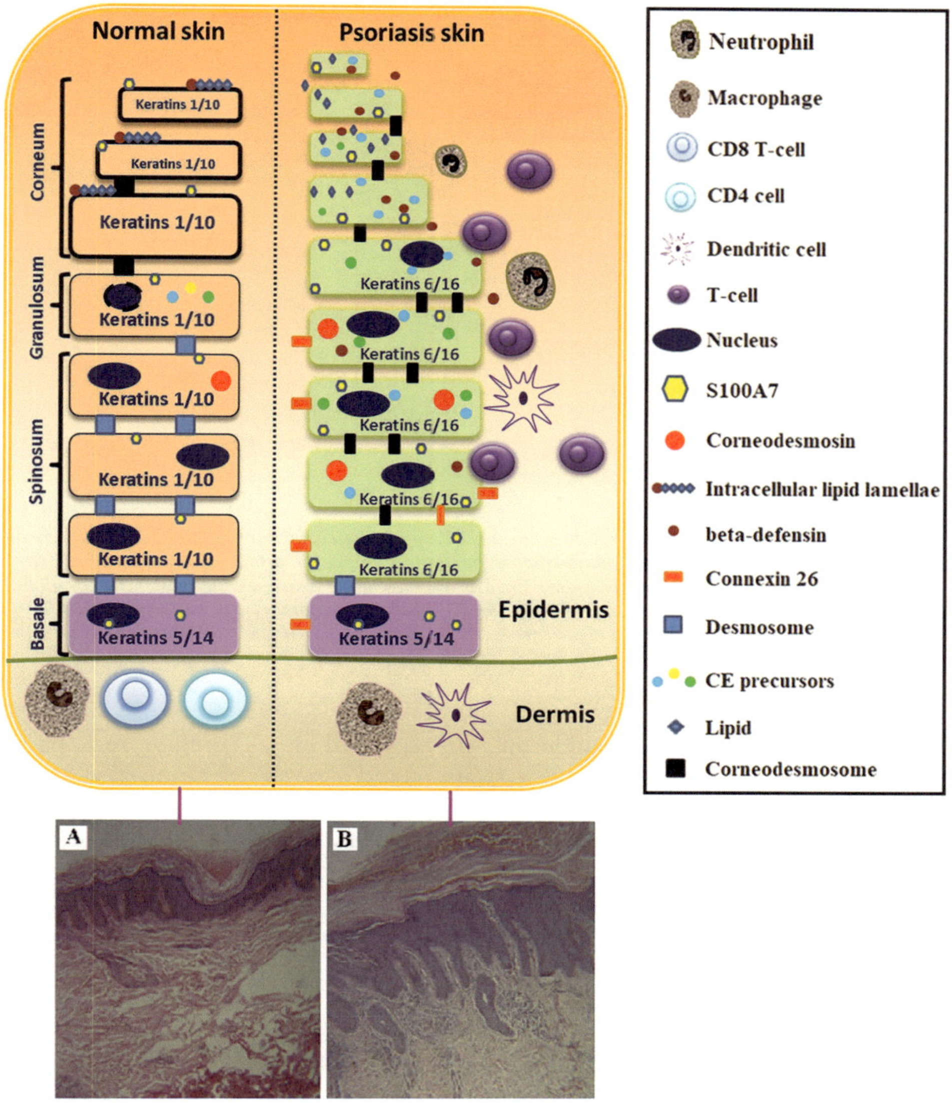

Figure 1.
Illustration of the epidermal layers of the normal skin and psoriatic skin including scaliness, hyperkeratosis, and neutrophil accumulation in the stratum corneum. A indicates immunohistology of normal skin, B indicates immunohistology of psoriatic skin.

2. Keratins involved in psoriasis

The hyperproliferation seemed to result from an increase in the number of transit amplifying cells, following depletion of the stem cell compartment [9, 26]. The differentiation state of epidermal KCs is reflected by the intricate expression pattern of keratins [27, 28]. Keratins are members of the large IF gene family [29] in all epithelia including the epidermis. Basal KCs express keratins (K) K5 and K14, which helps to maintain epidermal shape are replaced by differentiation keratin K1 and K10 [27], whereas in activated KCs, keratins K6, K16, and Keratin 17 (K17), which are distinct

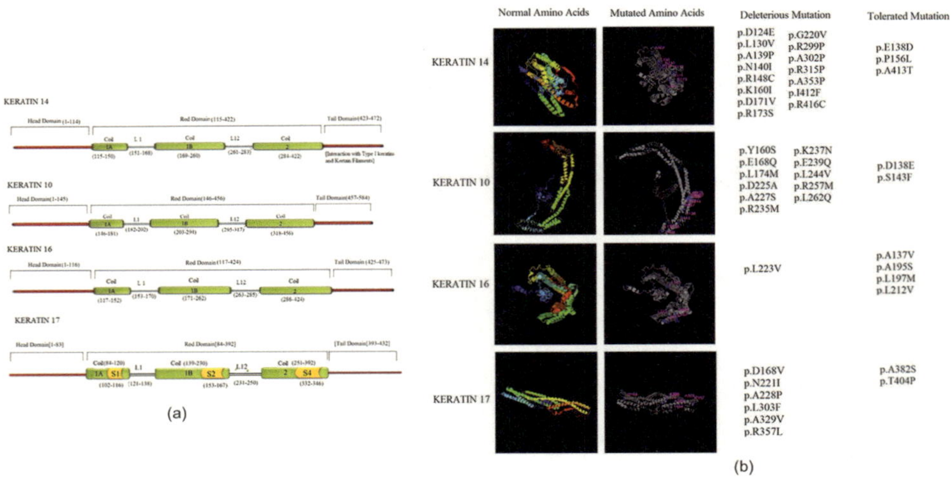

Figure 2.
Protein structure of epidermal and hyperproliferative keratins protein. (a) Schematic representation of secondary structure of all four keratins with their domain and sub domain. Whereas, S = peptide epitope; L = linker. (b) Region specific of 33 deleterious mutation localization. The left sides of the figures are the 3D structure of all four keratins CDS region. The right sides of the figures are the 3D structures of domains with mutated residues. The mutated residues are numbered according to their position on regions. The position of mutated amino acids (aa) on all four keratins and on CDS regions are provided [31].

from the keratins in the healthy epidermis, are expressed [30]. Therefore, keratins K6, K16, and K17 are usually referred to as activation- and hyperproliferation-associated keratins. There are predicted deleterious mutations were highly located in α-helical rod domain of keratins which forms coiled structure to these keratins, are important to maintain the structural integrity of the skin. Thus the genetic defects of basal keratin K14 and differentiation keratin K10 in skin might leads to express abnormal keratin pair which causes thickening of epidermis (acanthosis) in psoriasis (**Figure 2**).

2.1 Keratin 14

Keratin 5 and K14 pair are considered as a biochemical marker of mitotically active basal layers. This pairs are supports to maintain epidermal integrity as well as protects skin from mechanical stress. Interestingly, the K5/K14 pair is expressed in the basal layer of the epidermis, which contains epidermal stem cells and transient amplifying (TA) cells [32]. Many studies have showed that the level of K14 was considerably higher in lesional skin than in normal epidermis [33–35]. p53 activation promotes the expression of p21 and the repression of K14 during epidermal differentiation [36], whereas in psoriasis, there is downregulation of p53 [37] and also decreased Notch 1 expression [38] causes increase in K14 expression in psoriasis [39]. p75NTR is nearly absent in psoriatic KCs that are reportedly resistant to apoptosis, leads to increase TA cell turnover in psoriasis which leads to increase in K14 expression in psoriasis (**Figure 3**) [40].

2.2 Keratin 10

The epidermis is a stratified epithelium that regenerates permanently from the basal layer. K10 pair with K1 is considered as a major differentiation keratin [29]. Normally,the basal layer contains K14, K15, and K5, whereas suprabasal, postmitotic

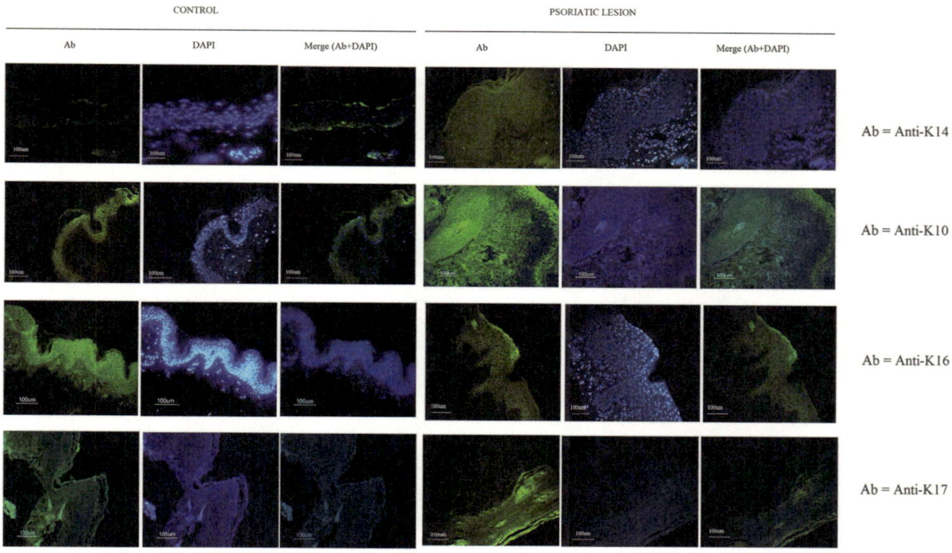

Figure 3.
Immunofluorescence analysis of keratins in control and lesional psoriatic skin. Immunofluorescence analysis of epidermal and hyperproliferative type I keratins in frozen skin sections from patients with psoriatic skin (×20 magnification, respectively), and nuclei were visualized with 4′-6-diamidino-2-phenylindole (DAPI). Bar = 100 μm. Ab = antibody [31].

cells switch to the expression of K1 and K10 [41, 42] is also involved in the control of cell proliferation [43]. Many studies have shown a downregulation of K1 and K10 [33–35] in psoriatic epidermis. This may be due to downregulation in E-cadherin expression [43], and increase in IL-22 [45–48] levels in psoriasis. Also c-fos protein in AP-1 transcription factor highly regulates a number of genes that are involved in KC differentiation were found to be reduced in psoriasis [49–52].

In psoriasis, defects in K10 expression leads to hyperproliferation of KCs by decreasing its inhibitory action on Rb phosphorylation, which leads to increased Cyclin D and E expression and also increased Phosho-Akt levels in psoriasis (**Figure 3**) [52].

2.3 Keratin 16

Keratin 16 expressions, reduces the fraction of cells in G1 while increasing that in S phase [52]. Many authors also shown an upregulation of K6 and K16 [33, 35, 54, 55] in psoriatic epidermis. Decrease expression of keratin 10 gene leads to hyperproliferation of basal cells, alterations in epidermal cell cycle by inducing cmyc, cyclin D1, 14-3-3σ, keratin 6 and keratin 16 [56]. Multiple transcription factors activated by the extracellular signals revealed the specific signals transduction mechanisms that respond to the corresponding growth factors and cytokines. For example, interleukin-1 (IL-1), present in healthy epidermis in inactive form [57], when released autocrinely, activates NFκB and C/EBPβ, thus initiating KC activation. Among the characteristics of activated KCs is the production of tumor necrosis factor-α (TNF-α) [58], which maintains activated NFκB and C/EBPβ. Activated KCs produce ligands of the EGF receptor that cause activation of AP1, such as transforming growth factor-α (TGF-α), amphiregulin and HB-EGF. Interestingly, all these cytokines and

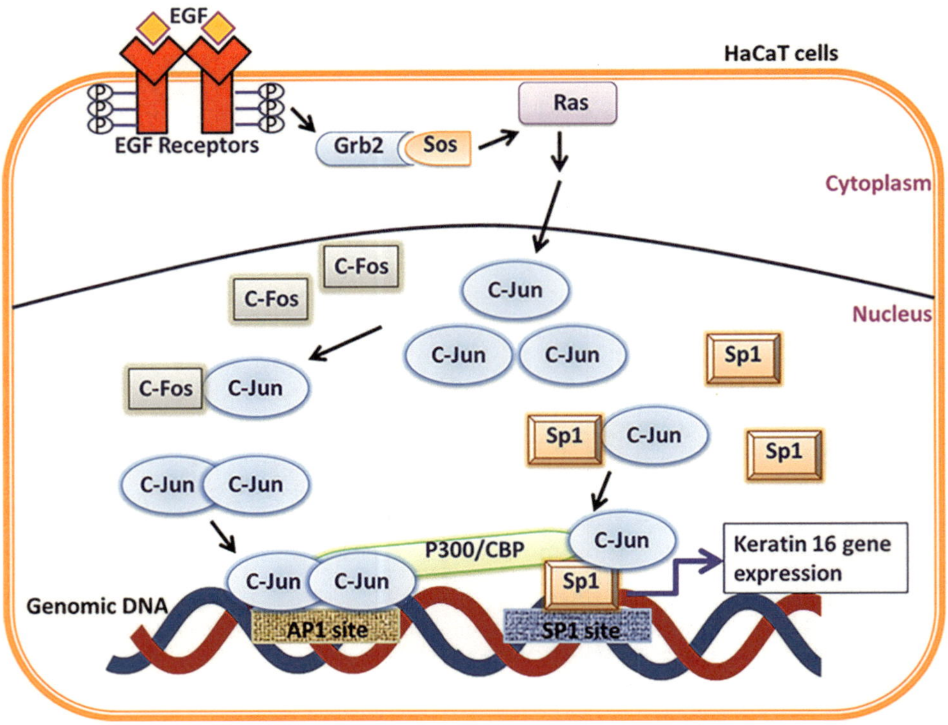

Figure 4.
Transcriptional regulation of the human keratin 16 gene in HaCaT cells.

growth factors IL-1, TNF-α, TGF-α and EGF, induce expression of the K16 genes, albeit through separate pathways [54, 59–61]. Study has shown that biosynthesis of AP1 protein (c-Jun and c-Fos) through Ras activation are actively participate in the transcriptional regulation for EGF which induced keratin 16 gene expression in KCs [62], this implies that EGF induces Keratin 16 expression in psoriasis (**Figure 4**).

2.4 Keratin 17

Keratin 17 (K17) is a type I intermediate filament mainly expressed in the basal cells of epithelial in hair follicles. As a complex cytoskeletal protein, K17 regulates a numereous biological processes in epithelial layer, including cell proliferation and growth, skin inflammation and hair follicle cycling. Abnormal expression of K17 is found in various diseases ranging from psoriasis to malignancies such as breast, cervical, oral squamous and gastric carcinomas [63, 64].

Many studies have showed the aberrant expression of K17 in psoriatic epidermis [35, 65, 66]. This aberrant expression is mainly due to interferon-γ (IFN-γ) produced by activated T cell [67]. Various inflammatory mediators like IFN-γ, IL-6, IL-17 A, IL-22 derived from T cells induced transcription of keratin K17 through STAT3- and ERK1/2-dependent mechanisms [64, 68, 69]. Thus, all these cytokines are involved in the induction of K17/T cell/cytokine autoimmune loop and play an important role in the progression of psoriasis [68].

3. Keratinocyte activation cycle (KAC)

Basal KC have two alternative pathways to end up. In normal skin, KCs undergo proliferation in basal layer and differentiation in both spinosus, granular layer, finally it end up as anucleate corneocytes in cornified layers. During all these process, various factors like calcium, retinoic acid, vitamin D3 and protein kinase C (PKC) activators are required to induce proliferation and differentiation in epidermis [70–74]. For proliferation and differentiation, Epidermal KCs required a pair of kertain proteins, for instance, in normal skin Keratin pair K5/K14 expressed in basal layer and K1/K10 are expressed in spinosus layer [75].

However, in pathological conditions like epidermal injury, cancer and psoriasis an alternative KCs pathway is get activated by inflammatory mediators. This alternative pathway disturbed normal proliferation and migrating phenotype in KCs [76, 77]. This alternative pathway is considered as a unusual cycle formed by the interaction of KCs-immunocytes, which is precisely elucidated as KC activation cycle [78]. This activation cycle begins with leakage of interleukin-1 beta (IL-1 β) from KC after any injury or disease condition. This inflammatory mediator initiate activation of KCs by changing the keratin pattern from K5/14 to K6/16 and firmly maintained by TNF-α and TGF-α [60, 61, 75, 79]. After any treatment or lesional healing stage, IFN-γ was released by KCs which act as a signal for healing process and also induces the expression of K17 [69, 80]. To normalize the healed skin, a transforming growth factor-β (TGF-β) synthesized from dermal fibroblasts were found to aid KCs phenotype by producing K5/14 keratin in basal layer (**Figure 5**) [81].

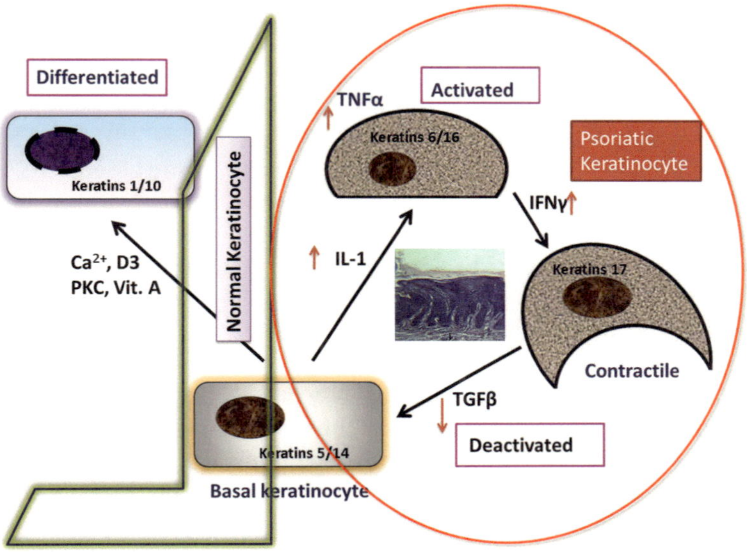

Figure 5.
The KC activation cycle. In normal KC, Basal layer produces K5 and K14 and differentiate to K1 and K10 with the help of ca2+, D3. Whereas in psoriatic KCs, K5 and K14 produce K6 and K16 by IL-1. TNF-α help to maintains activated KCs. Then, IFN-γ prompts K17 expression which stimulates KCs contractility. TGF-γ,a de-activating signal is not produced during psoriass, thereby hyperproliferation of epidermis in psoriasis. Symbol ↑ indicates increase in psoriasis; symbol ↓ indicates decrease in psoriasis.

3.1 Initiator of activation

The most common initiator of KC activation is IL-1. In pathological conditions like psoriasis, KC process and release IL-1, allowing the surrounding cells to perceive it [82–84]. The released IL-1 serves as a paracrine signal to dermal endothelial cells to become activated, express selectins, and slow down the circulating lymphocytes [85, 86]. IL-1 also serves as a chemoattractant for lymphocytes, causing them to extravasate and migrate to the site of lesion [87]. Furthermore, IL-1 is an activator of dermal fibroblasts, enhancing their migration, proliferation, and production of dermal extracellular matrix components [88]. IL-1 is also an autocrine signal that activates KC. IL-1 causes them to proliferate, become migratory, and express an activation-specific set of genes [76]. Thus, IL-1 initiates KC activation not only by triggering additional signaling events, but also by inducing directly the synthesis of K6/K16 in epidermal KC, and thus changing the composition of their cytoskeleton.

3.2 Maintenance of activation

TNF-α induced by IL-1 can maintain KCs in an activated state [75]. In psoriasis, a wide variety of cells produce TNF-α, primarily macrophages and monocytes but also epithelial cells including KCs [89]. TNF-α activates immune responses by inducing production of additional signaling molecules, cytokines, growth factors, their receptors, and adhesion proteins (e.g., amphiregulin, TGF-α, IL-1 α, IL-1 receptor antagonist, epidermal growth factor receptor (EGFR), and intercellular adhesion molecule (ICAM-1) [90]. In response to the activation of the EGFR, KCs proliferate, degrade components of the extracellular matrix, and become migratory [91].

3.3 The activated phenotype

Once activated, KCs synthesize additional signaling growth factors and cytokines including TGF-α IL-3, IL-6, IL-8, G-CSF, GM-CSF, and M-CSF [91, 92]. These signaling molecules produced by KCs act as paracrine signal to white blood cells, lymphocytes, fibroblasts, and endothelial cells in dermis. Apart from paracrine, it also acts as an autocrine signal for KCs in epidermis. Numerous cell surface proteins and integrins are also found to act as secondary moiety to activate epidermal KCs [93, 94].

3.4 The contractile keratinocyte

Psoriasis is associated with high levels of IFN-γ in epidermis [91]. IFN-γ strongly and specifically induced the promoter of the K17 (abnormal marker) gene. K17 is exceptional because it is not found in healthy interfollicular epidermis, but it is expressed in certain pathologic states, psoriasis [28]. The function of K17 in epidermis therefore may be to promote or allow KC contractility and/or frequent changes in shape [95]. Indeed, expression of K17 has been used to evaluate the course of treatment of psoriatic patients [63]. Due to failure, to resolve the deregulated inflammatory response in psoriasis leads to the persistent activation of KCs, which is characterized by prolonged K17 expression [13].

3.5 Back to normal basal phenotype

To revert to the basal cell phenotype, KCs need a signal. This signal comes from the dermal fibroblasts in the form of TGF-β. Cell kinetics study by Van Ruissen et al.

[96] clearly indicate that the TGF-β donot control KCs normal proliferation, but it controls the abnormal proliferation of KCs (antihyperproliferative). Whereas in psoriasis, the expression of TGF-β is low [97]. So the activation cycle is not reverted to normal basal phenotype, therefore hyperproliferation of KC takes place in psoriasis.

4. Methotrexate

MTX is the most commonly used systemic agent for psoriasis and, because it has been available for 35 years, most dermatologists are comfortable with its use. It is considered as an longstanding effective oral medication for the treatment of various types of psoriasis [98, 99]. Generally psoriasis treatment is mainly depends on the PASI score. For mild psoriasis patients, doctors prescribed topical therapy and phototherapy. For moderate to severe disease who have at least 5% of their skin covered with psoriasis are treated with oral medications like MTX, cyclosporine. [100]. Folate supplementation along with MTX reduces the incidence of megaloblastic anemia, hepatotoxicity, and gastrointestinal intolerance [101].

4.1 History

Anti-metabolites mimic substances required for normal biochemical reactions and thus interfere with normal functions of the cell, including cell division. They may masquerade as purines (e.g., azathioprine), pyrimidines (e.g., 5-flourouracil) and folic acid analogs essential for purine and pyrimidine synthesis, (e.g., MTX). Methotrexate, formerly known as aminopterin, has been widely used in the treatment of cancer and autoimmune diseases [102]. It was first developed in the 1940s when scientists were investigating the effects of folic acid on cancer, particularly childhood leukemia [103]. MTX is an analog of folic acid that inhibits cellular proliferation inducing folate coenzyme deficiencies [104]. When MTX was incidentally noted to improve psoriatic lesions in the 1960s it became clear that it possessed anti-inflammatory properties in addition to its antiproliferative effects [105–107]. Anti-inflammatory actions of MTX is accomplished by inhibiting dihydrofolate reductase which eventually diminishes the de novo synthesis of purines and pyrimidines and increases the catabolism of AMP and adenosine to IMP and inosine. Increased catabolism leads to accumulation of adenosine which confers anti-inflammatory effects of MTX [108].

4.2 Chemical structure of methotrexate

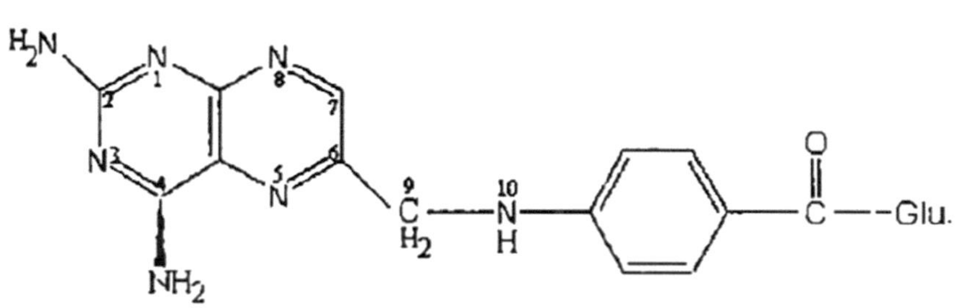

(2S)-2-[[4-[[2,4-bis (azanyl)pteridin-6-yl]methyl-methylamino]phenyl]carbonylamino] pentanedioic acid.

5. Clinical efficacy of methotrexate on psoriasis

Even though MTX has been used extensively for the treatment of psoriasis, so far its efficacy has not been supported by any clinical datas. A non-randomized controlled trial study done by our research team showed PASI 75 was achieved in 75% of psoriasis patients after 7.5 mg of MTX orally per week for a period of 12 weeks. PASI 75 is defined as a reduction from baseline PASI score of >75%. PASI 75 is used as the benchmark of primary end points in assessing therapies for psoriasis. Patients reaching PASI 75 represent very meaningful changes in psoriasis severity [109–112]. A randomized controlled clinical trial using 15 mg of MTX for 16 weeks in moderate to severe plaque has showed 60% of patients achieved a PASI-75 response (no significant difference, $P = 0.29$), [113, 114]. For safety consideration, MTX has found to be administered along with 5 mg of folic acid to minimize the serious toxicity include hematological disorder, hepatotoxicity and gastrointestinal toxicity, MTX has also affect lymphocytes and also cause autoimmune reaction at extreme usage [115–117]. But, several studies has shown that 5–10 mg of MTX cause less side-effect on liver of

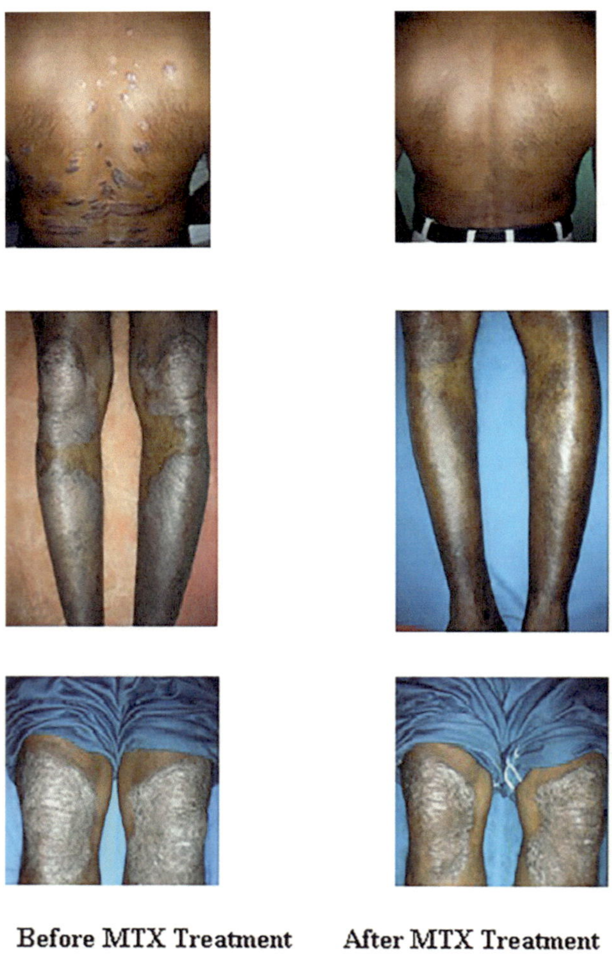

Figure 6.
Clinical efficacy of MTX on psoriatic patients.

psoriasis patients [118–121]. However more than 15 mg will cause severe side effects in psoriasis patients [121]. Clinical improvement of psoriatic patients before and after treatment of 7.5 mg of MTX per week for 12 weeks were depicted in (**Figure 6**).

Overall, the clinical data from our research study and also from other clinical trial has strongly supports that using low dose of MTX is well and safe for the treatment of moderate to severe psoriasis patients, and also frequent expert supervision along with laboratory monitoring is necessary.

6. Metabolic activity of methoxerate on psorisis

MTX mechanisms of action are likely to account for its antiproliferative and immunosuppressive effects [122, 123]. The key feature of psoriasis is KC hyperproliferation. MTX was found to induce maturation and inhibition of KC proliferation through its metabolic action of keratinocyte. The putative effects of MTX are listed below:

1. Reduction of cell proliferation

2. Increase of apoptosis of T cells

3. Increase of endogenous adenosine release

4. Alteration of expression of cellular adhesion molecules and

5. Influence on production of cytokines, humoral responses, and bone formation.

6.1 Effect of methotrexate on T cells

Evidence supports that activated T cells are key players in the immunopathogenesis of psoriasis. The following components involving T cells are considered crucial in the pathogenesis of psoriasis. Activated endothelium of psoriatic skin has shown adhesion molecules like E-selectin, CLA, ICAM-1 and ICAM-3, which promoted the activation of KCs and T-cells in psoriasis. Study by Sigmundsdottir et al. showed that treatment of 5–25 mg of MTX in 16 moderate to severe psoriasis patients has showed decreased E-selectin and CLA expression in psoriatic skin. Thus, the downregulation of peripheral Tcell-adhesion interaction by MTX in psoriasis patients implies its therapeutic action on psoriatic skin lesion [124]. Invitro flowcytometric and immunohistochemistry studies have shown that peripheral T cells were found to show less interaction with CLA and ICAM-1 after MTX administration 10^{-9} M to 10^{-5} M for 5 days. Follow-up experiments revealed that MTX suppression of CLA expression could be reversed by folinic acid (leucovorin) supplementation [123].

MTX has also target T cell by inducing cytolysis. Some studies has shown that MTX induce Tcell apoptosis in more sensitive manner [125–127]. MTX may induce cell death via free radical oxygen species. Phillips et al. [126] inhibited MTX induced T-cell death with the addition of the antioxidant glutathione and its precursor, Nacetylcysteine. Accumulating evidence suggests that MTX alters T-cell production of several cytokines, including IL-1, IL-2, IL-4, IL-8, INF-γ and TNF-α [128–131]. As a key element in psoriasis pathogenesis, the cytokine TNF-α was found at higher levels in psoriasis plaques and the synovial fluid of patients with psoriatic arthritis [129, 132, 133]. Associations between MTX and TNF-α levels have been observed since the 1990s. Studies by Seitz et al. [132], Neurath et al. [134] and Hildner et al. [135] found that MTX had reduced TNF-α production in the peripheral blood mononuclear cells (PBMCs) of psoriasis patients.

Action of MTX on reducing serum and synovial TNF-α has been widely established in both Psoriasis and rheumatoid arthritis patients showed its immunomodulatory effects [136–138]. Based on the stage and route of T-cell activation, it has been evident that MTX inhibits T-cell TNF-α production [129, 130, 135]. These all findings suggest that MTX can diminish TNF-α produced by activated T cells showed its immunomodulatory action.

6.2 Effects of methotrexate on endothelial cells

T-cell migration from the intravascular space into the dermis is a crucial step in the pathogenesis of psoriasis, and this process is dependent on interactions between endothelial cells and T cells. Endothelial expression of appropriate adhesion ligands such as E-selectin and ICAM-1, are necessary for successful T-cell adhesion and migration [124, 139]. Studies have shown that MTX treatment firmly decreased the CLA, ICAM-1 and E-selectin expression in the endothelial cells [24].
Histologically, hypervascularity is noted in psoriatic skin, which contributes to the grossly observed erythema. When used at the high dosages necessary for chemotherapy, MTX is capable of inhibiting angiogenesis. MTX exerted its therapeutic effects in psoriasis by inhibiting angiogenesis.In 2003 Yamasaki et al. [140] found that MTX had an inhibitory effect on endothelial cell growth. Two years later, in 2005, Yazici et al. [25] employed immunohistochemistry on lesional skin biopsies to study the effects of MTX on angiogenesis, reporting a statistically significant decrease in the endothelial marker CD31 after treatment with MTX.

Dendritic cells (DCs) are considered as a key player in the pathogenesis of psoriasis. Interplay between DCs, T-cells and cytokine are main and complex in psoriasis. DCs are well recognized has antigen-presenting cells (APC) in the skin. Any modulation in APC interaction with other cells may significantly influence development of psoriatic lesions. Many studies has showed that MTX showed its immunomodulatory effect by suppressing APCs activity [141, 142]. Recently, the use of T-cell targeted therapy confirmed the critical role of lymphocytes [143]. On the other hand, the clinical phenotype observed in psoriasis is mostly accounted for by several alterations in epidermal KCs [144].

7. Action of methotrexate on activated KC-immunocyte cycle in psoriasis

The epidermis is a multilayered epithelium consisting mainly of proliferating and differentiated, postmitotic KCs [145]. The latter derive from transit amplifying cells originating from stem cells that represent a restricted number of basal KCs [146, 147]. The proliferation and differentiation of epidermal KCs is regulated by a multitude of signaling cascades and transcription factors including Wnt/b-catenin [148], growth factors of the EGF and FGF family [149], TGF-β, members of the NFkB family [150], and c-Myc [151].

7.1 Activation and deactivation signals of KAC

In psoriasis, KCs undergo activation pathway. This activation process is governed by growth factors and cytokines, such IL-1, TNF-α, IFN-γ and TGF-β [78].

7.1.1 Interleukin-1

IL-1 is likely to be an important mediator in the initiation and maintenance of psoriatic plaques and may represent an attractive therapeutic target [152].

7.1.1.1 Interleukin-1 alpha

Our studies in IL-l α levels and its action in psoriasis had clearly showed that IL-l α level is reduced in psoriatic skin as well as in plasma [153], which was further supported by several studies [154–157]. Mechanism behind this reduction is mainly depend on the upstream level of nerve growth factor, a IL-1 α down-regulator [158, 159] in psoriasis.

The second messenger cyclic adenosine monophosphate (cAMP) has been regarded as a regulator for cell growth and proliferation [160]. The action of IL-l α is mainly depends on its phosphorylation by cyclic cAMP-dependent protein kinase. Thus, phosphorylation converts it into active form and enhanced its susceptibility to tryptic digestion, which may allow its release into the extracellular milieu [161]. Reduced cAMP levels has been reported in psoriasis [162]. This also could lead to reduced IL-l α levels in lesional skin biopsies.

Studies showed that MTX significantly increased IL-l α levels in plasma and skin biopsies of psoriasis patients. This may due to increase in the levels of cAMP by MTX through adenosine release [153, 163] and that led to an increase in IL-1 α level.

7.1.1.2 Interleukin-1 beta and caspase-1

Many studies have reported the importance of IL-1 β and caspase-1 (IL-1 β converting enzyme) in pathogenesis of psoriasis [153, 156, 157, 164]. Increased expression of IL-1 β in psoriatic epidermal cells, related to the activated KC-immunocyte in psoriasis. Psoriatic plaques express increased IL-1 β mRNA relative to non-lesional skin [161]. IL-1 β has been shown to induce the expression of adhesion molecules on various cell types and contributes to inflammatory responses. Activation of ERK, JNK, AP-1, and NFκB are leads to IL-1 β-induced ICAM-1 expression and leukocyte adhesion [165], thereby increase in ICAM-1 cause hyperproliferation of KC in psoriasis.

Normal KCs do not contain a biologically active form of caspases-1 [166], whereas in psoriatic epidermis, caspase-5 act as an upstream activator of caspase-1 [167]. Caspase-5 mRNA is induced by IFN-γ in vitro in both KCs and PBMCs and that this induction is most likely mediated through the NFκB pathway [168].

Mizutani et al. [169] found that IL-1 β levels in PBMC of psoriatic patients were decreased after 2 weeks of MTX treatment, due to suppression of KC paracrine system by MTX. Also, MTX effectively reduced IL-1 β levels in plasma and skin biopsies of psoriasis patients [153]. There are two possible mechanism of MTX decrease IL-1 β is elucidated above. One is direct mechanism and another one is indirect mechanism. The direct mechanism is as follows: MTX treatment inhibits the enzyme5-aminoimidazole-4-carboxamide ribonucleotide (AICAR) transformylase (ATIC), which leads to accumulation of the substrate AICAR. The increased AICAR inhibit the enzymes, AMP deaminase and adenosine deaminase, which are essential for the catabolism of AMP and adenosine. This inhibitory action eventually increased adenosine in circulation. Thus, increased extracellular adenosine firmly increased cAMP in skin which finally inhibits the production of proinflammatory cytokine IL-1 β [163].

The indirect mechanism of MTX on reducing IL-1 β levels in psoriasis is mainly depend on reduction of infiltration of lymphocytes and monocytes in psoriatic dermis [162, 170]. MTX also decreased g the circulating and systemic levels of IL-1 β, by blocking the binding of IL-1 β to its respective receptor on monocytes, lymphocytes and granulocytes [171]. Studies have shown that IL-l α down-regulates IL-1 β via prostaglandin E_2 synthesis [172]. Therefore increase in IL-1 α levels by MTX, definitely downregulates IL-1 β by above said mechanisms. Another mechanisms of MTX reduced IL-1 β, its action on caspase-1 expression in lesional skin biopsy. This may due to IFN-γ reduction by MTX [173, 174], which leads to decrease in caspase-5 expression that causes reduction in caspase-1 expression.

7.1.2 Tumor necrosis factor alpha

TNF-α is a pivotal proinflammatory cytokine of the innate immune response and a key for skin inflammation [175]. TNF-α induce the expression of adhesion molecule ICAM-1 on KC through the mediation of p55 and ICAM-1 induces the infiltration of MNCs in the dermis, which promotes the development and progression of psoriasis vulgaris [176]. Thereby it causes hyperproliferation in psoriasis.

Many studies have shown that plasma concentration of TNF-α was significantly higher in psoriatic patients compared to the control group [35, 177, 178]. Johansen [179] showed increased TNF-α protein expression, but similar TNF-α mRNA levels, in lesional compared with nonlesional psoriatic skin, this results showed that TNF-α is regulated posttranscriptionally. Increased activation of MAPK-activated protein kinase 2 (MK2) is responsible for the elevated and posttranscriptionally regulated TNF-α protein expression in psoriatic skin. IL-1 β also amplified TNF-α protein expression by causing activation of p38 MAPK and MK2.

Action of MTX to overwhelm TNF activity is by suppressing TNF-induced nuclear factor-κB activation in vitro, in part related to a reduction in the degradation and inactivation of an inhibitor of this factor, IκBα, and probably related to the release of adenosine [180]. Gerards et al. [130] showed that Adenosine or adenosine receptor agonists inhibit production of TNF-α. MTX reduces TNF-α level and also reduces the adhesion molecules like E-selctin and ICAM-1, thereby it reduces TNF-α induced hyperproliferation in psoriasis. Decrease in TNF-α by MTX shows its anti-proliferative and anti-inflammatory effects.

7.1.3 Interferon-γ

IFN-γ is believed to be an important mediator in psoriasis. Accumulated evidence from both in vivo and in vitro studies show that IFN-γ is a critical element in the induction of KC hyperproliferation in psoriasis [172, 181]. Abdallah et al. [182] showed that serum IFN-γ is a psoriasis severity and prognostic marker.

Some authors showed that serum IFN-γ levels in psoriatic patients were 15-fold and in blister fluid 17-fold higher than those in the control group. They correlated with the clinical severity of psoriasis expressed as PASI score [183–186]. In lesional skin, expression of IFN-γ is induced by some cytokines like IL-12, IL-18, and IL-23 are termed as IFN-γ stimulator [187]. Apart from above said stimulator, IL-7 also indirectly increased IFN-γ levels in both the psoriatic skin and serum of psoriatic patients. Inflammatory mediator IL-7 interact with both IL-2 and IL-12, which indirectly induced the synthesis of IFN-γ in psoriatic skin [188].

MTX treatment effectively reduced IFN-γ levels in serum and skin biopsy of psoriatic patients. This may due to the action of MTX on reducing serum IL-7 levels and is found to correlate with disease in RA patients [20]. Similar to this result, studies have shown that MTX decreases the expression of IFN-γ in RA patients [135, 136]. Adenosine or adenosine receptor agonists inhibit production of IFN-γ [130]. In 1990, Nesher and Moore [189] proposed that MTX might inhibit polyamine synthesis in monocytes, thereby polyamines failed to restore IFN-γ production.

As we discussed earlier in this chapter about the MTX action on T cell cytolysis, the same concept is applicable in this mechanism. The primary source of activated T cell is IFN-γ [127]. MTX induce the cytolysis of activated T-cell which directly reduced the IFN-γ in psoriasis. Invitro studies showed that inhibition of NFκB led to the complete blockade of extracellular IL-17A, IL-22, IFN-γ, and TNF-α production in CD4+ cells [190]. It is well known that MTX directly inhibit NFκB [191]. Thus, MTX declines IFN-γ levels by inhibiting NFκB in psoriatic skin which control the hyperproliferation of KCs.

7.1.4 Transforming growth factor-β1

In the skin, TGF-β has been found to inhibit the growth of KCs but stimulate the growth of fibroblasts [192]. Plasma TGF-β1 is considered as a biomarker of psoriasis activity and treatment efficacy [193].

Gene and protein expression of TGF-β1 in lesional skin biopsies was found to be reduced compared to nonlesional skin biopsies [35, 97, 193]. Reduction in TGF-β1 in psoriasis may be due to increase in activated Akt levels. Activated Akt inhibit the phosphorylation of Smad2/3, is essential for TGF-β1 production [194, 195]. IFN-γ and NF-kappaB induces the expression of Smad7, an antagonistic Smad, which prevents the interaction of Smad3 with the TGF-β receptor [196, 197] leading to TGF-β1 production. Other factors that can suppress TGF-β1 productions are Th1 cytokines like TNF-α, IL-1, IL-6 [196]. All these factors could have lead to reduction in TGF-β1 levels in psoriasis. Reduction in TGF-β1 leads to increase in proliferation of KCs in psoriasis. Adhesiveness of T lymphocytes to dermal microvascular endothelial cells can be blocked by TGF-β1, so reduction of its expression and function may contribute to lymphocyte infiltration into psoriatic plaques [198].

MTX treatment causes overexpression of protein and mRNA level of TGF-β1 in lesional skin biopsy. Possible mechanism of MTX is accompanied by decreasing Ras methylation in psoriasis. This hypomethylation is accompanied by a mislocalization of Ras to the cytosol and a 4-fold decrease in the activation of Akt [199]. Decrease in Akt may lead to Smad 3 activation, which in turn increase TGF-β1 expression. Also MTX reduces Th1 cytokines like IL-1, IFN-γ, TNF-α, IL-6 [111, 135, 136, 188] which may lead to increase in TGF-β1 expression. Increase in TGF-β1 expression induced inhibition of KCs and is characterized by reversible retention of proliferation, or stopping of cell division cycle in the G1 phase [96]. Moreover, TGF-β causes transcriptional induction of K5 and K14 keratin genes [81]. Thus, TGF-β promotes the basal cell phenotype in stratified epithelia such as the epidermis, and that the effects of TGF-β are not anti-proliferative, but merely anti-hyperproliferative [78].

7.2 Keratin changes in psoriatic skin after MTX action

The pathogenesis of psoriasis is mainly depend on KCs and immune cells interaction. These interaction causes changes in the epidermal layers which destined the healthy skin to lesional psoriatic skin is critical one. Due to the epidermal change, acanthosis is caused by disruption in the transition of KC to anucleate corneocytes. This disrupts transition leads to hyperproliferation and immatured differentiation of KC in psoriasis. Thus, an alternate or regenerative pathway is activated by abnormal immune response along with abnormal keratins in psoriatic epidermis [200].

7.2.1 Keratin 14

K14 is an important IF expressed in the basal KCs which decide the fate of epidermis by protecting it from any mechanical or chemical disturbances. Normallay, basal layer contains epidermal stem cells and TA cells that proliferate into KCs. The epidermal stem cells and TA cells expressed keratin K5/K14 which destined the cells to proliferate into KC [32].

In psoriatic skin biopsy, K14 expression was considerably higher than in normal epidermis [33–35]. However, MTX reduced the expressions of K14 in lesional skin biopies by increasing Phosphorylated form of p53 expression [201]. Studies have shown that p53 enhance the notch signaling [202], which leads to modulation and normalization of K14 expression to K10 differentiation marker. Thus, decrease in K14 expression leads to reduction in cell proliferation, decrease in phospho-Akt levels, increase in activated Notch1 levels, and increase in levels of KC differentiation markers [39] and also increased in p21 and p27 levels, which are known to be direct targets of Notch1 signals. Activation of p21 and p27 leads to cell cycle arrest [191, 203] which leads to inhibition of hyperproliferating KCs in psoriasis.

7.2.2 Keratin 10

When mitotically active basal epidermal KCs withdrawn from the cell cycle are committed to terminal differentiation, they switch off K14 expression and induce the expression of K10 [27]. K10 are the major structural proteins of the epidermis and belong to the large family of IF proteins [29, 41, 42]. K10 is also involved in the control of cell proliferation [43]. Decreased K10 protein and gene expression were observed in lesional psoriatic skin biospies [33–35]. Subsequently, hyperproliferation of KCs in psoriasis is mainly depend on the expression of K10. The possible mechanism is as follows, decrease in differentiation marker K10 leads to increased phosphorylation of Rb protein, which leads to increased epidermal cell cycle proteins, Cyclin D and E. The increased epidermal cell cycle proteins activate the phosphorylation of antiapoptotic protein Akt. Thus activation of Akt by decreased K10 leads to hyperproliferation of KCs in psoriasis [52].

E-cadherin is specific markers expressed in the endothelial cells are important for differentiation process. MTX promptly increased E-cadherin expression [201] which deliberately causes extracellular calcium concentration-dependent KC differentiation by increasing K10 in psoriatic skin. IL-22 which is considered to have an inhibitory effect on the expression of K10 [205], is reduced by MTX in psoriasis patients [206]. Also MTX increase c-fos expression which activate AP-1 transcription factor regulates K10 expression [207]. Thus MTX action on K10 expression proves the controlled differentiation in psoriatic KC.

The main therapeutic action of MTX is inhibiting DNA methylation by interfering folate metabolism [207]. Studies have shown that inhibition of DNA methylation directly increased transcription of K10 gene [208]. This shows the therapeutic action of MTX on psoriatic skin.

7.2.3 Keratin 16

Keratin 16 expressions, reduces the fraction of cells in G1 while increasing that in S phase [53]. Many authors also shown an upregulation of K6 and K16 [33–35] in psoriatic epidermis. Action of MTX on reducing Keratin 16 protein and mRNA expression in lesional skin biopsies is interesting. Ras signaling is also induces K16 in psoriasis. The action of MTX in decreasing K16 level is depends on the enzyme isoprenylcysteine carboxyl methyltransferase (Icmt). Inhibition of Icmt by MTX, indicates the link between antifolates and Ras. Icmt inhibition leads to decrease in carboxyl methylation of Ras [199], which induces EGF. Induced EGF directly decreased K16 expression. Overall mechanism indicates the action of MTX on K16 reduction. Apart from this, MTX also inhibits the IL-1, TNF-α levels [135, 153, 169], which also might leads to decrease in K16 expression in psoriasis. All these leads to inhibition of cell proliferation in psoriasis. Decrease in Keratin 16 by MTX indicates the strong anti-proliferative effect of MTX.

7.2.4 Keratin K17

Keratin K17, the myoepithelial keratin, which is not expressed in normal skin except for hair follicles, sweat and sebaceous glands and basal cells of the interfollicular epidermis in the scalp, is over-expressed in psoriatic epidermis [209, 210]. Keratin 17 is considered as a therapeutic target and marker of anti-psoriatic therapies used for the treatment of psoriasis [63, 64].

MTX substantially reduced abnormal K17 protein and gene expression in psoriasis by reducing circulatory inflammatory mediators like IL-22 [205] and IL-6 levels [111] in psoriasis patients. Many studies in Rheumatoid Arthritis patients showed that the production of IL-17 at the mRNA level and IFN-γ were reduced after MTX treatment [35, 135, 211]. Altogether MTX reduces K17 expression by decreasing IFN-γ inducers. Decrease in Keratin 17 by MTX indicates its therapeutic efficacy which helps to maintain the normal phenotype in KC.

8. Conclusion

When we put all these data and review together, we attain at a consistent outline for the action of keratins, growth factors and cytokines in psoriasis. MTX has been used as a effective agent in the treatment of psoriasis from the decades of 1960s. But still its mechanisms of clearing psoriatic remains ill-defined. In conclusion, we strongly thought that MTX inhibits the hyperproliferation of KCs by decreasing the levels of IL-1 and caspases-1 (activating signals), TNF-α, IFN-γ and by increasing deactivation signal through various effective pathway. Also it efficiently regulate abnormal keratins by upregulating K10 and downregulating K14, K16 and K17, thereby maintaining the normal phenotype in KC (**Figure 7**). Mutation in keratins filaments were also observed in psoriasis [31]. Thereby, understanding keratin functions and related regulatory mechanisms will help to design new therapeutic interventions for keratin-related skin diseases. We strongly concluded that MTX roles on controlling the KC-immunocyte cycle by activating important keratins and deactivating abnormal kertains showed its well-organized therapeutic effect in psoriasis patients.

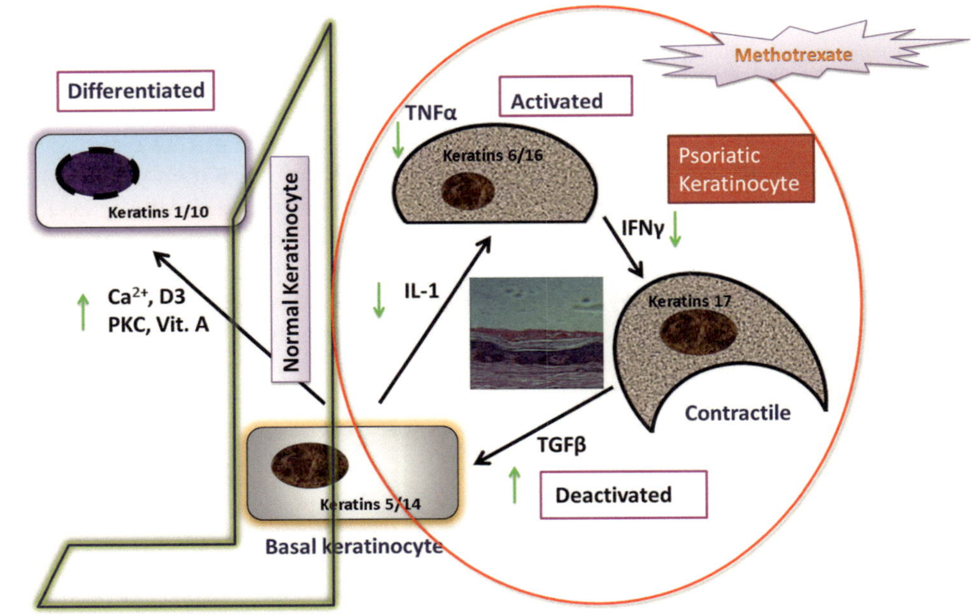

Figure 7.
Effect of MTX on KC activation cycle. MTX normalizing or reversing the phenotype of psoriatic KC but altering the inflammatory mediators as well as keratin proteins in KCs. Symbol ↑ indicates increase in psoriasis; symbol ↓ indicates decrease in psoriasis.

Acknowledgements

We thank all patients who have assisted for all our studies.

Conflict of interests

The authors declare that they have no conflict of interests.

Abbreviation

KAC	keratinocyte activation cycle
KC	keratinocyte
IL	interleukin
MTX	methotrexate
TNF	tumor necrosis factor
IFN	interferon
TGF	transforming growth factor
K14	keratin 14
K10	keratin 10
K16	Keratin 16
K17	keratin 17

Author details

Tamilselvi Elango[1,2*], Anburaj Jeyaraj[2,3], Haripriya Dayalan[4], Pushpa Gnanaraj[5], Xinghui Li[2*] and Xuejun Zhang[1*]

1 Institute and Department of Dermatology, The First Affiliated Hospital, Anhui Medical University, Hefei, China

2 Tea Research Institute, College of Horticulture, Nanjing Agricultural University, Nanjing, China

3 Department of Biotechnology, Karpagam Academy of Higher Education, Tamilnadu, India

4 Department of Biotechnology, Rajalakshmi Engineering College, Chennai, Tamilnadu, India

5 Department of Dermatology, Apollo Speciality Hospitals, Tamilnadu, India

*Address all correspondence to: tami24684@gmail.com, lxh@njau.edu.cn and ayzxj@vip.sina.com

References

[1] Van Onselen J. Psoriasis in general practice. Nursing Standard. 1998;**12**:32-33

[2] Ortonne JP. Etiology and pathogenesis of psoriasis. The British Journal of Dermatology. 1996;**135**(49S):1-5

[3] Zenz R, Eferl R, Kenner L, et al. Psoriasis-like skin disease and arthritis caused by inducible epidermal deletion of Jun proteins. Nature. 2005;**437**(7057):369-375

[4] Nickoloff BJ, Nestle FO. Recent insights into the immunopathogenesis of psoriasis provide new therapeutic opportunities. Journal of Clinical Investigation. 2004;**113**(12):1664-1675

[5] Hussein MR, Al-Badaiwy ZH, Guirguis MN. Analysis of p53 and bcl-2 protein expression in the non-tumorigenic, pre-tumorigenic and tumorigenic keratinocyte hyper proliferative lesions. Journal of Cutaneous Pathology. 2004;**31**(10):643-651

[6] Gottlieb AB. Infliximab for psoriasis. Journal of the American Academy of Dermatology. 2003;**49**(Suppl. 2):S112-S117

[7] Carlen LM et al. Proteome analysis of skin distinguishes acute guttate from chronic plaque psoriasis. Journal of Investigative Dermatology. 2005;**124**(1):63-69

[8] Zhou X et al. Novel mechanisms of T-cell and dendritic cell activation revealed by profiling of psoriasis on the 63,100-element oligonucleotide array. Physiological Genomics. 2003;**13**(1):69-78

[9] Waikel RL, Kawachi Y, Waikel PA. Deregulated expression of c-Myc depletes epidermal stem cells. Nature Genetics. 2001;**28**:165-168

[10] Zibert JR, Lovendorf MB, Litman T, et al. MicroRNAs and potential target interactions in psoriasis. Journal of Dermatological Science. 2010;**58**:177-185

[11] Pasquinelli AE. NON-CODING RNA MicroRNAs and their targets: Recognition, regulation and an emerging reciprocal relationship. Nature Reviews. Genetics. 2012;**13**:271-282

[12] Selbach M, Schwanhausser B, Thierfelder N, et al. Widespread changes in protein synthesis induced by microRNAs. Nature. 2008;**455**:58-63

[13] Coronnello C, Benos PV. ComiR: Combinatorial microRNA target prediction tool. Nucleic Acids Research. 2013;**41**:W159-W164

[14] Lindsay MA. microRNAs and the immune response. Trends in Immunology. 2008;**29**:343-351

[15] Baumjohann D, Ansel KM. MicroRNA-mediated regulation of T helper cell differentiation and plasticity. Nature Reviews Immunology. 2013;**13**:666-678

[16] Ichihara A, Jinnin M, Yamane K, et al. microRNA-mediated keratinocyte hyperproliferation in psoriasis vulgaris. The British Journal of Dermatology. 2011;**165**:1003-1010

[17] de Cid R, Riveira-Munoz E, Zeeuwen PL, et al. Deletion of the late cornified envelope LCE3B and LCE3C genes as a susceptibility factor for psoriasis. Nature Genetics. 2009;**41**(2):211-215

[18] Zhang XJ, Huang W, Yang S, et al. Psoriasis genome-wide association

study identifies susceptibility variants within LCE gene cluster at 1q21. Nature Genetics. 2009;**41**(2):205-210

[19] Lane EB, McLean WH. Keratins and skin disorders. Journal of Pathology. 2004;**204**(4):355-366

[20] Herman S, Zurgil N, Langevitz P, et al. Methotrexate selectively modulates TH1/TH2 balance in active rheumatoid arthritis patients. Clinical and Experimental Rheumatology. 2008;**26**:317-323

[21] Bonish B, Jullien D, Dutronc Y, et al. Overexpression of CD1d by keratinocytes in psoriasis and CD1d-dependent IFN-gamma production by NK-T cells. Journal of Immunology. 2000;**165**(7):4076-4085

[22] Sigmundsdóttir H, Gudjónsson JE, Jónsdóttir I, Lúdvíksson BR, Valdimarsson H. The frequency of CLA+ CD8+ T cells in the blood of psoriasis patients correlates closely with the severity of their disease. Clinical and Experimental Immunology. 2001;**126**(2):365-369

[23] Saleh A, Abuhilal M, Cheung B. Methotrexate in psoriasis: From A to Z. Journal of the Turkish Academy of Dermatology. 2010;**4**:04101r

[24] Dahlman-Ghozlan K, Ortonne JP, Heilborn JD, Stephansson E. Altered tissue expression pattern of cell adhesion molecules, ICAM-1, E-selectin and VCAM-1, in bullous pemphigoid during methotrexate therapy. Experimental Dermatology. 2004;**13**(2):65-69

[25] Yazici AC, Tursen U, Apa DD, et al. The changes in expression of ICAM-3, Ki-67, PCNA, and CD31 in psoriatic lesions before and after methotrexate treatment. Archives of Dermatological Research. 2005;**297**(6):249-255

[26] Johnston A, Gudjonsson JE, Sigmundsdottir H, et al. The anti-inflammatory action of methotrexate is not mediated by lymphocyte apoptosis, but by the suppression of activation and adhesion molecules. Clinical Immunology. 2005;**114**(2):154-163

[27] Fuchs E, Green H. Changes in keratin gene expression during terminal differentiation of the keratinocyte. Cell. 1980;**19**:1033-1042

[28] Moll R, Moll I, Franke WW. Differences of expression of cytokeratin polypeptides in various epithelial skin tumors. Archives of Dermatological Research. 1984;**276**(6):349-363

[29] Hesse M, Magin TM, Weber K. Genes for intermediate filament proteins and the draft sequence of the human genome: Novel keratin genes and a surprisingly high number of pseudogenes related to keratin genes 8 and 18. Journal of Cell Science. 2001;**114**:2569-2575

[30] Machesney M, Tidman N, Waseem A, et al. Activated keratinocytes in the epidermis of hypertrophic scars. The American Journal of Pathology. 1998;**152**(5):1133-1141

[31] Elango T, Sun J, Zhu C, et al. Mutational analysis of epidermal and hyperproliferative type I keratins in mild and moderate psoriasis vulgaris patients: A possible role in the pathogenesis of psoriasis along with disease severity. Human Genomics. 2018;**12**(1):27

[32] Coulombe PA, Kopan R, Fuchs E. Expression of keratin K14 in the epidermis and hair follicle: Insights into complex programs of differentiation. Journal of Cell Biology. 1989;**109**:2295-2312

[33] Castelijns FA, Gerritsen MJ, van Vlijmen-Willems IM, et al. Proliferation is the main epidermal target in the

treatment of psoriatic plaques with once daily application of tacalcitol ointment. Acta Dermato-Venereologica. 1999;**79**(2):111-114

[34] Thewes M, Stadler R, Korge B, Mischke D. Normal psoriatic epidermis expression of hyperproliferation-associated keratins. Archives of Dermatological Research. 1991;**283**(7):465-471

[35] Elango T, Thirupathi A, Subramanian S, Dayalan H, Gnanaraj P. Methotrexate normalized keratinocyte activation cycle by overturning abnormal keratins as well as deregulated inflammatory mediators in psoriatic patients. Clinica Chimica Acta. 2015;**451**(Pt B):329-337

[36] Cai BH, Hsu PC, Hsin IL, et al. p53 acts as a co-repressor to regulate keratin 14 expression during epidermal cell. PLoS One. 2012;**7**(7):e41742

[37] Xiaolian G, Elisabet N, Philip JC. Effect of narrow-band ultraviolet B phototherapy on p63 and microRNA (miR-21 and miR-125b) expression in psoriatic epidermis. Acta Dermato-Venereologica. 2011;**91**:392-397(6)

[38] Thélu J, Rossio P, Favier B. Notch signaling is linked to epidermal cell differentiation level in basal cell carcinoma, psoriasis and wound healing. BMC Dermatology. 2002;**2**:7

[39] Alam H, Sehgal L, Kundu ST, et al. Novel function of keratins 5 and 14 in proliferation and differentiation of stratified epithelial cells. Molecular Biology of the Cell. 2011;**22**(21):4068-4078

[40] Truzzi F, Marconi A, Atzei P, et al. p75 neurotrophin receptor mediates apoptosis in transit-amplifying cells and its overexpression restores cell death in psoriatic keratinocytes. Cell Death and Differentiation. 2011;**18**(6):948-958

[41] Herrmann H, Hesse M, Reichenzeller M, Aebi U, Magin TM. Functional complexity of intermediate filament cytoskeletons: From structure to assembly to gene ablation. International Review of Cytology. 2003;**223**:83-175

[42] Hesse M, Zimek A, Weber K, Magin TM. Comprehensive analysis of keratin gene clusters in humans and rodents. European Journal of Cell Biology. 2004;**83**:19-26

[43] Reichelt J, Furstenberger G, Magin TM. Loss of keratin 10 leads to mitogen-activated protein kinase (MAPK) activation, increased keratinocyte turnover, and decreased tumor formation in mice. Journal of Investigative Dermatology. 2004;**123**(5):973-981

[44] Li ZX, Ji FP, Peng ZH, Wang K. Expression of E-cadherin, beta-catenin and cyclin D1 in epidermal skin lesions of patients with active psoriasis vulgaris. Nan Fang Yi Ke Da Xue Xue Bao. 2008;**28**(4):545-547

[45] Boniface K, Bernard FX, Garcia M, et al. IL-22 inhibits epidermal differentiation and induces proinflammatory gene expression and migration of human keratinocytes. Journal of Immunology. 2005;**174**(6):3695-3702

[46] Wolk K, Witte E, Wallace E, et al. IL-22 regulates the expression of genes responsible for antimicrobial defense, cellular differentiation, and mobility in keratinocytes: A potential role in psoriasis. European Journal of Immunology. 2006;**36**(5):1309-1323

[47] Sa SM, Valdez PA, Wu J, et al. The effects of IL-20 subfamily cytokines on reconstituted human epidermis suggest potential roles in cutaneous innate defense and pathogenic adaptive

immunity in psoriasis. Immunology. 2007;**178**:2229-2240

[48] Nograles KE, Zaba LC, Guttman-Yassky E, et al. Th17 cytokines interleukin (IL)-17 and IL-22 modulate distinct inflammatory and keratinocyte-response pathways. The British Journal of Dermatology. 2008;**159**(5):1092-1102

[49] Johansen C, Kragballe K, Henningsen J, et al. 1a,25-dihydroxyvitamin D3 stimulates activator protein 1 DNA-binding activity by a phosphoinositol 3-kinase/Ras/MEK/extracellular signal regulated kinase 1/2 and c-jun N-terminal kinase 1-dependent increase in cfos,fra1, and c-jun expression in human keratinocytes. Journal of Investigative Dermatology. 2003;**120**:561-570

[50] Schmuth M, Elias PM, Hanley K, et al. The effect of LXR activators on AP-1 proteins in keratinocytes. Journal of Investigative Dermatology. 2004;**123**:41-48

[51] Eckert RL, Crish JF, Efimova T, et al. Regulation of involucrin gene expression. Journal of Investigative Dermatology. 2004;**123**:13-22

[52] Basset-Seguin N, Escot C, Moles JP, et al. C-fos and c-jun proto-oncogene expression is decreased in psoriasis: An in situ quantitative analysis. Journal of Investigative Dermatology. 1991;**97**:672-678

[53] Paramio JM, Casanova ML, Segrelles C, et al. Modulation of cell proliferation by cytokeratins K10 and K16. Molecular and Cellular Biology. 1999;**19**(4):3086-3094

[54] Komine M, Rao LS, Kaneko T, et al. Inflammatory vs. proliferative processes in the epidermis: Tumor necrosis factor alpha induces K6b keratin synthesis through a transcriptional complex containing NFkB and C/EBPb. Journal of Biological Chemistry. 2000;**275**:32077-32088

[55] van de Kerkhof PCM, Jorn Bovenschen H, et al. In vivo effects of topical anti-psoriatic treatments on cutaneous inflammation, epidermal proliferation and keratinisation. Current Drug Therapy. 2007;**2**:21-26

[56] Reichelt J, Magin TM. Hyperproliferation, induction of c-Myc and 14-3-3σ, but no cell fragility in keratin-10-null mice. Journal of Cell Science. 2002;**115**:2639-2650

[57] Kupper TS. The activated keratinocyte: A model for inducible cytokine production by non-bone marrow-derived cells in cutaneous inflammatory and immune responses. Journal of Investigative Dermatology. 1990;**94**:146S-150S

[58] Barker JN, MacDonald DM. Cutaneous lymphocyte trafficking in the inflammatory dermatoses. British Journal of Dermatology. 1992;**126**:211-215

[59] Pittelkow MR, Lindquist PB, Abraham RT, et al. Induction of transforming growth factor-alpha expression in human keratinocytes by phorbol ester. Journal of Biological Chemistry. 1989;**264**:5164-5171

[60] Jiang CK, Magnaldo T, Ohtsuki M, et al. Epidermal growth factor and transforming growth factor alpha specifically induce the activation- and hyperproliferation associated keratins 6 and 16. Proceedings of the National Academy of Sciences. 1993;**90**:6786-6790

[61] Komine M, Rao LS, Freedberg IM, et al. Interleukin-1 induces transcription of keratin K6 in human epidermal keratinocytes. Journal of Investigative Dermatology. 2001;**116**:330-338

[62] Wang YN, Chang WC. E Induction of disease-associated keratin 16 gene expression by epidermal growth factor is regulated through cooperation of transcription factors Sp1 and c-Jun. Journal of Biological Chemistry. 2003;**278**(46):45848-45857

[63] de Jong EMGJ, van Vlijmen IMMJ, et al. Keratin 17: A useful marker in anti-psoriatic therapies. Archives of Dermatological Research. 1991;**283**(7):480-482

[64] Vogel U, Denecke B, Sergey M, et al. Transcriptional activation of psoriasis-associated cytokeratin K17 by interferon-γ Analysis of γ-interferon activation sites. European Journal of Biochemistry. 1995;**227**:143-149

[65] de Jong EMG, Ferrier CM, de Zwart A, et al. Effects of topical treatment with budesonide on parameters for epidermal proliferation, keratinization and inflammation in psoriasis. Journal of Dermatological Science. 1995;**9**:185-194

[66] Baker BS, Swain AF, Fry L, Valdmarsson H. Epidermal T lymphocytes and HLA-DR expression in psoriasis. British Journal of Dermatology. 1984;**110**:555-564

[67] Jiang CK, Flanagan S, Ohtsuki M, et al. Disease-activated transcription factor: Allergic reactions in human skin cause nuclear translocation of stat-91 and induce synthesis of keratin K17 molecular effects of T lymphocytes on the regulation of keratin gene expression. A cluster of five nuclear proteins regulates keratin gene transcription. Molecular and Cellular Biology. 1994;**14**(7):4759-4769

[68] Zhang W, Dang E, Shi X, Jin L, Feng Z, et al. The pro-inflammatory cytokine IL-22 up-regulates Keratin 17 expression in keratinocytes via STAT3 and ERK1/2. PLoS One. 2012;**7**(7):e40797

[69] Komine M, Freedberg IM, Blumenberg M. Regulation of epidermal expression of keratin K17 in inflammatory skin diseases. Journal of Investigative Dermatology. 1996;**107**(4):569-575

[70] Hennings H, Michael D, Cheng C. Calcium regulation of growth and differentiation of mouse epidermal cells in culture. Cell. 1980;**19**(1):245-254

[71] Fuchs E, Green H. Regulation of terminal differentiation of cultured human keratinocytes by vitamin A. Cell. 1981;**25**(3):617-625

[72] Hosomi J, Hosoi J, Abe E, et al. Regulation of terminal differentiation of cultured mouse epidermal cells by 1 alpha,25-dihydroxyvitamin D3. Endocrinology. 1983;**113**(6):1950-1957

[73] Parkinson EK, Pera MF, Emmerson A. "Differential effects of complete and second-stage tumor promoters in normal but not transformed human and mouse keratinocytes," Carcinogenesis. 1984;**5**(8):1071-1077

[74] Eckert RL, Crish JF, Robinson NA. The epidermal keratinocyte as a model for the study of gene regulation and cell differentiation. Physiological Reviews. 1997;77(2):397-424

[75] Darmon M, Blumenberg ML. Molecular Biology of the Skin: The Keratinocyte. San Diego: Academic Press; 1993

[76] Nickoloff BJ, Turka LA. Keratinocytes: Key immunocytes of the integument. The American Journal of Pathology. 1993;**143**(2):325-331

[77] Tomic-Canic M, Komine M, Freedberg IM, et al. Epidermal signal transduction and transcription factor activation in activated keratinocytes. Journal of Dermatological Science. 1998;**17**(3):167-181

[78] Freedberg IM, Tomic-Canic M, Komine M, et al. Keratins and the keratinocyte activation cycle. Journal of Investigative Dermatology. 2001;**116**(5):633-640

[79] Ma S, Rao L, Freedberg IM, Blumenberg M. Transcriptional control of K5, K6, K14, and K17 keratin genes by AP-1 and NF-kappaB family members. Gene Expression. 1997;**6**(6):361-370

[80] Jiang CK, Flanagan S, Ohtsuki M. Disease-activated transcription factor: Allergic reactions in human skin cause nuclear translocation of STAT-91 and induce synthesis of keratin K17. Molecular and Cellular Biology. 1994;**14**(7):4759-4769

[81] Jiang CK, Tomic-Canic M, Lucas DJ, et al. TGF beta promotes the basal phenotype of epidermal keratinocytes: Transcriptional induction of K#5 and K#14 keratin genes. Growth Factors. 1995;**12**(2):87-97

[82] Zepter K, Haffner A, De Soohoo LF, et al. Induction of biologically active IL-1 beta converting enzyme and mature IL-1 beta in human keratinocytes by inflammatory and immunologic stimuli. Journal of Immunology. 1997;**159**(12):6203-6208

[83] Corsini E, Primavera A, Marinovich M, Galli CL. Selective induction of cell associated interleukin-1alpha in murine keratinocytes by chemical allergens. Toxicology. 1998;**129**(2-3):193-200

[84] Murphy JE, Robert C, Kupper TS. Interleukin-1 and cutaneous inflammation: A crucial link between innate and acquired immunity. Journal of Investigative Dermatology. 2000;**114**(3):602-608

[85] Romero LI, Zhang DN, Herron GS, Karasek MA. Interleukin-1 induces major phenotypic changes in human skin microvascular endothelial cells. Journal of Cellular Physiology. 1997;**173**(1):84-92

[86] Wyble CW, Hynes KL, Kuchibhotla J, et al. TNF alpha and IL-1 upregulate membrane-bound and soluble E-selectin through a common pathway. Journal of Surgical Research. 1997;**73**(2):107-112

[87] Santamaria Babi LF, Moser R, Perez Soler MT. Migration of skin-homing T cells across cytokine-activated human endothelial cell layers involves interaction of the cutaneous lymphocyte-associated antigen (CLA), the very late antigen-4 (VLA-4), and the lymphocyte function associated antigen-1 (LFA-1). Journal of Immunology. 1995;**154**(4):1543-1550

[88] Maas-Szabowski N, Fusenig NE. Interleukin-1-induced growth factor expression in postmitotic and resting fibroblasts. Journal of Investigative Dermatology. 1996;**107**(6):849-855

[89] Kolde G, Schulze-Osthoff K, Meyer H, et al. Immunohistological and immunoelectron microscopic identification of TNF alpha in normal human and murine epidermis. Archives of Dermatological Research. 1992;**284**(3):154-158

[90] Griffiths TW, Griffiths CE, Voorhees JJ. Immunopathogenesis and immunotherapy of psoriasis. Dermatologic Clinics. 1995;**13**(4):739-749

[91] Nickoloff BJ, Griffiths CE, Barker JN. The role of adhesion molecules, chemotactic factors, and cytokines in

inflammatory and neoplastic skin disease. Journal of Investigative Dermatology. 1990;**94**(Suppl. 6):151S-157S

[92] Kupper TS. Role of epidermal cytokines. In: Oppenheim JJ, Shevach EM, editors. Immunophysiology. The Role of Cells and Cytokines in Immunity and Inflammation. London and New York: Oxford University Press; 1990. pp. 285-305

[93] Marinkovich MP, Lunstrum GP, Keene DR, et al. The dermal-epidermal junction of human skin contains a novel laminin variant. Journal of Cell Biology. 1992;**119**(3):695-703

[94] Burgeson RE. Type VII collagen, anchoring fibrils, and epidermolysis bullosa. Journal of Investigative Dermatology. 1993;**101**(3):252-255

[95] Troyanovsky SM, Leube RE, Franke WW. Characterization of the human gene encoding cytokeratin 17 and its expression pattern. European Journal of Cell Biology. 1992;**59**(1):127-137

[96] van Ruissen F, van Erp PEJ, de Jongh GJ. Cell kinetic characterization of growth arrest in cultured human keratinocytes. Journal of Cell Science. 1994;**107**(8):2219-2228

[97] Nockowski P, Szepietowski JC, Ziarkiewicz M. Serum concentrations of transforming growth factor beta 1 in patients with psoriasis vulgaris. Acta Dermatovenerologica Croatica. 2004;**12**(1):2-6

[98] Ryan TJ, Vickers HR, Salem SN, et al. The treatment of psoriasis with folic acid antagonist. The British Journal of Dermatology. 1964;**76**:555-564

[99] Boffa M, Chalmers R. Methotrexate for psoriasis. Clinical and Experimental Dermatology. 1996;**21**:399-408

[100] Bright R. Methotrexate in the treatment of psoriasis. Cutis. 1999;**64**:332-334

[101] Strober BE, Menon K. Folate supplementation during methotrexate therapy for patients with psoriasis. Journal of the American Academy of Dermatology. 2005;**53**:652-659

[102] Gubner R, August S, Ginsberg V. Therapeutic suppression of tissue reactivity. II. Effect of aminopterin in rheumatoid arthritis and psoriasis. The American Journal of the Medical Sciences. 1951;**221**:176-182

[103] Ward JR. Historical perspective on the use of methotrexate for the treatment of rheumatoid arthritis. Journal of Rheumatology. 1985;**12**:3-6

[104] Cronstein BN. Molecular therapeutics: Methotrexate and its mechanism of action. Arthritis and Rheumatism. 1996;**39**:1951-1960

[105] Lynch JP III, McCune J. Immunosuppressive and cytotoxic pharmacotherapy for pulmonary disorders. American Journal of Respiratory Critical Care Medicine. 1997;**155**:395-420

[106] Kremer JM. Methotrexate update. Scandinavian Journal of Rheumatology. 1996;**25**(6):341-344

[107] Goodman TA, Polisson RP. Methotrexate: Adverse reactions and major toxicities. Rheumatic Diseases Clinics of North America. 1994;**20**:513-528

[108] Chan ES, Cronstein BN. Methotrexate—how does it really work? Nature Reviews Rheumatology. 2010;**6**:175-178

[109] Griffiths CEM, Clark CM, Chalmers RJG, et al. A systematic review

of treatments for severe psoriasis. Health Technology Assessment. 2000;**4**(40):1-125

[110] Callis KP, Chadha A, Vaishnaw A, et al. Reduction of CD45RO+ effector T lymphocytes is not observed in the treatment of psoriasis with methotrexate. Journal of Investigative Dermatology. 2002;**119**:244 (abstract 220)

[111] Elango T, Dayalan H, Subramanian S, Gnanaraj P, Malligarjunan H. Serum interleukin-6 levels in response to methotrexate treatment in psoriatic patients. Clinica Chimica Acta. 2012;**413**(19-20):1652-1656

[112] Elango T, Dayalan H, Gnanaraj P, Malligarjunan H, Subramanian S. Impact of methotrexate on oxidative stress and apoptosis markers in psoriatic patients. Clinical and Experimental Medicine. 2014;**14**(4):431-437

[113] Heydendael VM, Spuls PI, Opmeer BC, et al. Methotrexate versus cyclosporine in moderate-to-severe chronic plaque psoriasis. The New England Journal of Medicine. 2003;**349**(7):658-665

[114] Sandhu K, Kaur I, Kumar B, et al. Efficacy and safety of cyclosporine versus methotrexate in severe psoriasis: A study from north India. Journal of Dermatology. 2003;**30**(6):458-463

[115] Gawkrodger DJ. On behalf of the Therapy Guidelines and Audit Subcommittee of the British Association of Dermatologists. Current management of psoriasis. Journal of Dermatological Treatment. 1997;**8**:27-55

[116] Said S, Jeffes EW, Weinstein GD. Methotrexate. Clinics in Dermatology. 1997;**15**(5):781-797

[117] Roenigk HH Jr, Auerbach R, Maibach HI. Methotrexate in psoriasis: Revised guidelines. Journal of the American Academy of Dermatology. 1988;**19**(1 pt1):145-156

[118] Roenigk HH Jr, Auerbach R, Maibach HI, et al. Methotrexate in psoriasis: Consensus conference. Journal of the American Academy of Dermatology. 1998;**38**(3):478-485

[119] Dogra S, Krishna V, Kanwar AJ. Efficacy and safety of systemic methotrexate in two fixed doses of 10. Clinical and Experimental Dermatology. 2012;**37**(7):729-734

[120] Yeo CM, Chong VH, Earnest A. Prevalence and risk factors of methotrexate hepatoxicity in Asian patients with psoriasis. World Journal of Hepatology. 2013;**5**(5):275-280

[121] Zachariae H. Have methotrexate-induced liver fibrosis and cirrhosis become rare? A matter for reappraisal of routine liver biopsies. Dermatology. 2005;**211**(4):307-308

[122] Kremer JM. Methotrexate treatment of rheumatic diseases: Can we do better? Arthritis and Rheumatism. 2008;**58**:3279-3282

[123] Wessels JA, Huizinga TW, Guchelaar HJ. Recent insights in the pharmacological actions of methotrexate in the treatment of rheumatoid arthritis. Rheumatology (Oxford). 2008;**47**:249-255

[124] Sigmundsdottir H, Johnston A, Gudjonsson JE, et al. Methotrexate markedly reduces the expression of vascular E-selectin, cutaneous lymphocyte-associated antigen and the numbers of mononuclear leucocytes in psoriatic skin. Experimental Dermatology. 2004;**13**(7):426-434

[125] Jeffes EW III, McCullough JL, Pittelkow MR, et al. Methotrexate

therapy of psoriasis: Differential sensitivity of proliferating lymphoid and epithelial cells to the cytotoxic and growth-inhibitory effects of methotrexate. Journal of Investigative Dermatology. 1995;**104**(2):183-188

[126] Phillips DC, Woollard KJ, Griffiths HR. The anti-inflammatory actions of methotrexate are critically dependent upon the production of reactive oxygen species. British Journal of Pharmacology. 2003;**138**(3):501-511

[127] Herman S, Zurgil N, Deutsch M. Low dose methotrexate induces apoptosis with reactive oxygen species involvement in T lymphocytic cell lines to a greater extent than in monocytic lines. Inflammation Research. 2005;**54**(7):273-280

[128] Magari K, Miyata S, Nishigaki F. Differential effects of FK506 and methotrexate on inflammatory cytokine levels in rat adjuvant-induced arthritis. Journal of Rheumatology. 2003;**30**(10):2193-2200

[129] Partsch G, Steiner G, Leeb BF. Highly increased levels of tumor necrosis factor-alpha and other proinflammatory cytokines in psoriatic arthritis synovial fluid. Journal of Rheumatology. 1997;**24**(3):518-523

[130] Gerards AH, de Lathouder S, de Groot ER. Inhibition of cytokine production by methotrexate. Studies in healthy volunteers and patients with rheumatoid arthritis. Rheumatology (Oxford, England). 2003;**42**(10):1189-1196

[131] Barsig J, Yam G, Lehner MD, Beume R. Methotrexate treatment suppresses local cytokine and chemokine production in rat adjuvant arthritis. Drugs under Experimental and Clinical Research. 2005;**31**(1):7-11

[132] Seitz M, Loetscher P, Dewald B, et al. Methotrexate action in rheumatoid arthritis: Stimulation of cytokine inhibitor and inhibition of chemokine production by peripheral blood mononuclear cells. British Journal of Rheumatology. 1995;**34**(7):602-609

[133] Partsch G, Wagner E, Leeb BF, et al. T cell derived cytokines in psoriatic arthritis synovial fluids. Annals of the Rheumatic Diseases. 1998;**57**(11):691-693

[134] Neurath MF, Hildner K, Becker C et al. "Methotrexate specifically modulates cytokine production by T cells and macrophages in murine collagen-induced arthritis (CIA): A mechanism for methotrexate-mediated immunosuppression". Clinical and Experimental Immunology. 1999;**115**(1):42-55

[135] Hildner K, Finotto S, Becker C, et al. Tumor necrosis factor (TNF) production by T cell receptor primed T lymphocytes is a target for low dose methotrexate in rheumatoid arthritis. Clinical and Experimental Immunology. 1999;**118**(1):137-146

[136] Constantin A, Loubet-Lescoulie P, Lambert N, et al. Antiinflammatory and immunoregulatory action of methotrexate in the treatment of rheumatoid arthritis: Evidence of increased interleukin-4 and interleukin-10 gene expression demonstrated in vitro by competitive reverse transcriptase polymerase chain reaction. Arthritis and Rheumatism. 1998;**41**(1):48-57

[137] Dolhain RJ, Tak PP, Dijkmans BA, et al. Methotrexate reduces inflammatory cell numbers, expression of monokines and of adhesion molecules in synovial tissue of patients with rheumatoid arthritis. British Journal of Rheumatology. 1998;**37**(5):502-508

[138] Kraan MC, Reece RJ, Barg EC, et al. Modulation of inflammation and metalloproteinase expression in synovial tissue by leflunomide and methotrexate in patients with active rheumatoid arthritis. Findings in a prospective, randomized, double-blind, parallel design clinical trial in thirty-nine patients at two centers. Arthritis and Rheumatism. 2000;**43**(8):1820-1830

[139] Bouma MG, van den Wildenberg FA, Buurman WA. Adenosine inhibits cytokine release and expression of adhesion molecules by activated human endothelial cells. The American Journal of Physiology. 1996;**270**(2Pt1):C522-C529

[140] Yamasaki E, Soma Y, Kawa Y, Mizoguchi M. Methotrexate inhibits proliferation and regulation of the expression of intercellular adhesion molecule-1 and vascular cell adhesion molecule-1 by cultured human umbilical vein endothelial cells. The British Journal of Dermatology. 2003;**149**(1):30-38

[141] Morhenn VB, Orenberg EK, Kaplan J, et al. Inhibition of a Langerhans cell mediated immune response by treatment modalities useful in psoriasis. Journal of Investigative Dermatology. 1983;**81**(1):23-27

[142] Liu HN, Wong CK. In vitro immunosuppressive effects of methotrexate and azathioprine on Langerhans cells. Archives of Dermatological Research. 1997;**289**(2):94-97

[143] Griffiths CE. T-cell-targeted biologicals for psoriasis. Current Drug Targets. Inflammation and Allergy. 2004;**3**(2):157-161

[144] Wrone-Smith T, Mitra RS, Thompson CB, et al. Keratinocytes derived from psoriatic plaques are resistant to apoptosis compared with normal skin. The American Journal of Pathology. 1997;**151**(5):1321-1329

[145] Watt FM, Hogan BL. Out of Eden: Stem cells and their niches. Science. 2000;**287**:1427-1430

[146] Taylor G, Lehrer MS, Jensen PJ, et al. Involvement of follicular stem cells in forming not only the follicle but also the epidermis. Cell. 2000;**102**(4):451-461

[147] Oshima H, Rochat A, Kedzia C, et al. Morphogenesis and renewal of hair follicles from adult multipotent stem cells. Cell. 2001;**104**(2):233-245

[148] Huelsken J, Vogel R, Erdmann B, et al. β-Catenin controls hair follicle morphogenesis and stem cell differentiation in the skin. Cell. 2001;**105**(4):533-545

[149] Werner S, Smola H. Paracrine regulation of keratinocyte proliferation and differentiation. Trends in Cell Biology. 2001;**11**(4):143-146

[150] Kaufman CK, Fuchs E. It's got you covered. NF-kappaB in the epidermis. Journal of Cell Biology. 2000;**149**(5):999-1004

[151] Arnold I, Watt FM. c-Myc activation in transgenic mouse epidermis results in mobilization of stem cells and differentiation of their progeny. Current Biology. 2001;**11**(8):558-568

[152] Mee JB, Cork M, di Giovineb FS, et al. Interleukin-1: A key inflammatory mediator in psoriasis? Cytokine. 2006;**33**(2):72-78

[153] Tamilselvi E, Haripriya D, Hemamalini M, Pushpa G, Swapna S. Association of disease severity with IL-1 levels in methotrexate-treated psoriasis patients. Scandinavian Journal of Immunology. 2013;**78**(6):545-553

[154] Takematsu H, Terui K, Ohkohchi H, et al. Interleukin-1-like activity in horny layer extracts: Decreased activity in scale extracts of psoriasis and sterile dermatoses. Dermatologica. 1986;**172**:236

[155] Takematsu H, Tagam H. Lack of correlation interleukin 1 levels between interleukin 6 in psoriatic lesional skin. Tohoku Journal of Experimental Medicine. 1994;**172**:243-252

[156] Yoshinaga Y, Higaki M, Terajima S. Detection of inflammatory cytokines in psoriatic skin. Archives of Dermatological Research. 1995;**287**:158-164

[157] Debets R, Hegmans JP, Croughs P, et al. The IL-1 system in psoriatic skin. IL-1 antagonist sphere of influence in lesional psoriatic epidermis. Journal of Immunology. 1997;**158**(2955):± 63

[158] Fantini F, Magnoni C, Bracci-Laudiero L, Pincelli C. Nerve growth factor is increased in psoriatic skin. Journal of Investigative Dermatology. 1995;**105**:854-855

[159] Pincelli C. Nerve growth factor and keratinocytes: A role in psoriasis. European Journal of Dermatology. 2000;**10**(2):85-90

[160] Ockenfels HM, Nussbaum G, Schneck B, et al. The effect of cyclosporin A and FK 506 on the cAMP content in psoriatic keratinocytes. Skin Pharmacology and Physiology. 1996;**9**(4):281-288

[161] Kobayashi Y, Appella E, Yamada M, et al. Phosphorylation of Intracellular Precursors of Human IL-1. Journal of Immunology. 1988;**14**:2279

[162] Barrera P, Boerbooms AM, Demacker PN, et al. Circulating concentrations and production of cytokines and soluble receptors in rheumatoid arthritis patients: Effects of a single dose Methotrexate. British Journal of Rheumatology. 1994;**33**:1017-1024

[163] Stamp LK, Hazlett J, Roberts RL, et al. Adenosine receptor expression in rheumatoid synovium: A basis for methotrexate action. Arthritis Research & Therapy. 2012;**14**:138

[164] Debets R, Hegmans JP, Troost RJ, et al. Enhanced production of biologically active interleukin-1a and interleukin-1b by psoriatic epidermal cells ex vivo: Evidence of increased cytosolic interleukin-1b levels and facilitated interleukin-1 release. European Journal of Immunology. 1995;**25**:1624-1630

[165] Yang CM, Luo SF, Hsieh HL, et al. Interleukin-1beta induces ICAM-1 expression enhancing leukocyte adhesion in human rheumatoid arthritis synovial fibroblasts: Involvement of ERK, JNK, AP-1, and NF-kappaB. Journal of Cellular Physiology. 2010;**224**(2):516-526

[166] Pietrzak AT, Zalewska A, Chodorowska G, et al. Invited critical review: Cytokines and anticytokines in psoriasis. Clinica Chimica Acta. 2008;**394**:7-21

[167] Martinon F, Tschopp J. Inflammatory caspases and inflammasomes: Master switches of inflammation. Cell Death and Differentiation. 2007;**14**:10-22

[168] Salskov-Iversen ML, Johansen C, Kragballe K. Caspase-5 expression is upregulated in lesional psoriatic skin. Journal of Investigative Dermatology. 2011;**131**(3):670-676

[169] Mizutani H, Ohmoto Y, Mizutani T, et al. Role of increased production of monocytes TNF-alpha, IL-1beta and IL-6 in psoriasis: Relation to focal

infection, disease activity and responses to treatments. Journal of Dermatological Science. 1997;**14**(2):145-153

[170] Chang DM, Weinblatt ME, Schur PH. The effects of methotrexate on interleukin 1 in patients with rheumatoid arthritis. Journal of Rheumatology. 1992;**19**:1678-1682

[171] Brody M, Böhm I, Bauer R. Mechanism of action of methotrexate: Experimental evidence that methotrexate blocks the binding of interleukin 1 beta to the interleukin 1 receptor on target cells. European journal of clinical chemistry. 1993;**31**(10):667-674

[172] Beta-Csorgo Z, Hammerberg C, Voorhees JJ, Cooper KD. Intralesional T-lymphocyte activation as a mediator of psoriatic hyperplasia. Journal of Investigative Dermatology. 1995;**105**:89S-894S

[173] Dinarello CA, Ikejima T, Warner SJ, et al. Interleukin 1 induces interleukin 1. I. Induction of circulating interleukin 1 in rabbits in vivo and in human mononuclear cells in vitro. Journal of Immunology. 1987;**139**:1902

[174] Thirupathi A, Elango T, Subramanian S, Gnanaraj P. Methotrexate regulates Th-1 response by suppressing caspase-1 and cytokines in psoriasis patients. Clinica Chimica Acta. 2016;**453**:164-169

[175] Bradley JR. TNF-mediated inflammatory disease. Journal of Pathology. 2008;**214**:149-160

[176] Shifa Z, Junping L, Yakun W, et al. Expressions of TNF receptors, ICAM-1 and LFA-1 in lesional skin of psoriasis vulgaris. Chinese Journal of Dermatology. 1998;**31**(2):84-86

[177] Mussi A, Bonifati C, Carducci M, et al. Serum TNF-alpha levels correlate with disease severity and are reduced by effective therapy in plaque-type psoriasis. Journal of Biological Regulators and Homeostatic Agents. 1997;**11**(3):115-118

[178] Chodorowska G. Plasma concentrations of IFN-gamma and TNF-alpha in psoriatic patients before and after local treatment with dithranol ointment. Journal of the European Academy of Dermatology and Venereology. 1998;**10**(2):147-151

[179] Johansen C, Funding AT, Otkjaer K, et al. Protein expression of TNF-alpha in psoriatic skin is regulated at a posttranscriptional level by MAPK-activated protein kinase 2. Journal of Immunology. 2006;**176**(3):1431-1438

[180] Majumdar S, Aggarwal BB. Methotrexate suppresses NfkappaB activation through inhibition of IkappaBalpha phosphorylation and degradation. Journal of Immunology. 2001;**167**:2911-2920

[181] Christophers E. The immunopathology of psoriasis. International Archives of Allergy and Immunology. 1996;**110**:199-206

[182] Abdallah MA, Abdel-Hamid MF, Kotb AM, Mabrouk EA. Serum interferon-gamma is a psoriasis severity and prognostic marker. Cutis. 2009;**84**(3):163-168

[183] Uyemura K, Yamamura M, Fivenson DF, Modlin RL. The cytokine network in lesional and lesion-free psoriatic skin is characterized by a T-helper type 1 cell-mediated response. Journal of Investigative Dermatology. 1993;**101**:701-705

[184] Schlaak JF, Buslau M, Jochum W, et al. T cells involved in psoriasis vulgaris belong to the Th1 subset. Journal of Investigative Dermatology. 1994;**102**:145-149

[185] El Barnawi NY, Ciasuddin ASM, Ziu MM, Singh M. Serum cytokine levels in psoriasis vulgaris. British Journal of Biomedical Science. 2001;**58**:40-44

[186] Arican O, Aral M, Sasmaz S, et al. Serum levels of TNF-alpha, IFN-gamma, IL-6, IL-8, IL-12, IL-17, and IL-18 in patients with active psoriasis and correlation with disease severity. Mediators of Inflammation. 2005;**5**:273-279

[187] Piskin G, Koomen CW, Picavet D. Ultraviolet-B irradiation decreases IFN-γ and increases IL-4 expression in psoriatic lesional skin in situ and in cultured dermal T cells derived from these lesions. Experimental Dermatology. 2003;**12**:172-180

[188] Bonifati C, Trento E, Cordiali-Fei P, et al. Increased interleukin-7 concentrations in lesional skin and in the sera of patients with plaque-type psoriasis. Clinical Immunology and Immunopathology. 1997;**83**:41-44

[189] Nesher G, Moore TL. The in vitro effects of methotrexate on peripheral blood mononuclear cells. Modulation by methyl donors and spermidine. Arthritis and Rheumatism. 1990;**33**:954-959

[190] Kagami S, Rizzo HL, Lee JJ, et al. Circulating Th17, Th22, and Th1 cells are increased in psoriasis. Journal of Investigative Dermatology. 2010;**130**(5):1373-1383

[191] Rangarajan A, Talora C, Okuyama R, et al. Notch signaling is a direct determinant of keratinocyte growth arrest and entry into differentiation. The EMBO Journal. 2001;**20**(13):3427-3436

[192] Cutroneo KR. TGF-beta-induced fibrosis and SMAD signaling: Oligo decoys as natural therapeutics for inhibition of tissue fibrosis and scarring. Wound Repair and Regeneration. 2007;**15**(1):S54-S60

[193] Flisiak I, Porebski P, Flisiak R, Chodynicka B. Plasma transforming growth factor beta1 as a biomarker of psoriasis activity and treatment efficacy. Biomarkers. 2003;**8**(5):437-443

[194] Conery AR, Cao Y, Thompson EA, et al. Akt interacts directly with Smad3 to regulate the sensitivity to TGF-beta induced apoptosis. Nature Cell Biology. 2004;**6**(4):366-372

[195] Song K, Wang H, Krebs T, Danielpour D. Novel roles of Akt and mTOR in suppressing TGF-b/ALK5-mediated Smad3 activation. The EMBO Journal. 2006;**25**:58-69

[196] Ulloa L, Doody J, Massagué J. Inhibition of transforming growth factor-beta/SMAD signaling by the interferon-gamma/STAT pathway. Nature. 1999;**397**(6721):710-713

[197] Bitzer M, von Gersdorff G, Liang D, et al. A mechanism of suppression of TGF-beta/SMAD signaling by NF-kappa B/RelA. Genes & Development. 2000;**14**(2):187-197

[198] Cai JP, Falanga V, Taylor JR, Chin YH. Transforming growth factor beta receptor binding and function are decreased in posriatic dermal endothelium. Journal of Investigative Dermatology. 1996;**106**:225-231

[199] Winter-Vann AM, Kamen BA, Bergo MO, et al. Targeting Ras signaling through inhibition of carboxyl methylation: An unexpected property of Methotrexate. Proceedings of the National Academy of Sciences. 2003;**100**(11):6529-6534

[200] Simpson CL, Patel DM, Green KJ. Deconstructing the skin: Cytoarchitectural determinants of epidermal morphogenesis. Nature

Reviews. Molecular Cell Biology. 2011;**12**:565-580

[201] Huang WY, Yang PM, Chang YF, Marquez VE, Chen CC. Methotrexate induces apoptosis through p53/p21-dependent pathway and increases E-cadherin expression through downregulation of HDAC/EZH2. Biochemical Pharmacology. 2011;**81**(4):510-517

[202] Yugawa T, Handa K, Narisawa-Saito M, Ohno S, Fujita M, Kiyono T. Regulation of Notch1 gene expression by p53 in epithelial cells. Molecular and Cellular Biology. 2007;**27**(10):3732-3742

[203] Sriuranpong V, Borges MW, Ravi RK, et al. Notch signaling induces cell cycle arrest in small cell lung cancer cells. Cancer Research. 2001;**61**(7):3200-3205

[204] Miyoshi K, Takaishi M, Nakajima K, et al. Stat3 as a therapeutic target for the treatment of psoriasis: A clinical feasibility study with STA-21, a Stat3 inhibitor. Journal of Investigative Dermatology. 2011;**131**(1):108-117

[205] Meephansan J, Ruchusatsawat K, Sindhupak W, Thorner PS, Wongpiyabovorn J. Effect of methotrexate on serum levels of IL-22 in patients with psoriasis. European Journal of Dermatology. 2011;**21**(4):501-504

[206] Spurlock CF, Aune ZT, Tossberg JT, et al. Increased sensitivity to apoptosis induced by methotrexate is mediated by JNK. Arthritis and Rheumatism. 2011;**63**(9):2606-2616

[207] Neradil J, Pavlasova G, Veselska R. New mechanisms for an old drug; DHFR- and non-DHFR-mediated effects of methotrexate in cancer cells. Klinická Onkologie. 2012;**2**:S87-S92

[208] Paradisi A, Pasquariello N, Barcaroli D, Maccarrone M. Anandamide regulates keratinocyte differentiation by inducing DNA methylation in a CB1 receptor-dependent manner. Journal of Biological Chemistry. 2008;**283**(10):6005-6012

[209] Leigh IM, Navsaria H, Purkis PE, et al. Keratins (K16 and K17) as markers of keratinocyte hyperproliferation in psoriasis in vivo and in vitro. The British Journal of Dermatology. 1995;**133**:501-511

[210] Fu M, Wang G. Keratin 17 as a therapeutic target for the treatment of psoriasis. Journal of Dermatological Science. 2012;**67**(3):161-165

[211] Li Y, Jiang L, Zhang S, Yin L, et al. Methotrexate attenuates the Th17/IL-17 levels in peripheral blood mononuclear cells from healthy individuals and RA patients. Rheumatology International. 2012;**32**(8):2415-2422

Section 3

Treatment of Psoriasis

Chapter 7

Topical Moisturisers for the Management of Psoriasis Vulgaris

Dalibor Mijaljica, Fabrizio Spada and Ian P. Harrison

Abstract

The aim of this chapter is to provide an overview of basic and tailored topical moisturisers and discuss how and why they form the backbone for the management of psoriasis. Our discussion begins by describing the main characteristics of psoriasis and by indicating how alterations in the skin's integrity and barrier function contribute to the initial development of psoriasis and subsequent changes in psoriasis phenotype. Next, we address the evolution of topical moisturisers to ever more sophisticated and beneficial products, and describe the key biophysical effects exerted on the psoriatic skin by their active ingredients, as well as the myriad benefits offered by fundamental and specialty ingredients. Furthermore, we delineate how topical moisturiser formulation modalities can help to improve compromised skin barrier function and to alleviate the symptoms of psoriasis, cosmetically and/or therapeutically as well as discuss the associated concerns and challenges encountered along the way.

Keywords: active, excipient, formulation modality, ingredient, management, basic moisturiser, tailored moisturiser, psoriatic plaque, skin barrier

1. Introduction

As a common and complex skin condition (Section 1.1), the root causes of psoriasis begin inside our body [1], making it far more than just skin deep. The fact that psoriasis affects the skin's hydration, barrier structure, function and integrity (Section 1.2) [2] means that a combination of several management strategies (Section 1.3) is usually required in order to alleviate associated symptoms [3, 4]. Topical moisturisers (Section 1.4) represent *the* first-line defence strategy that forms the backbone of psoriasis management by reducing and relieving both dryness and the associated itch-scratch cycle, enhancing skin hydration, and strengthening barrier function by influencing its subsequent repair and recovery [5–7] and thus, improving underlying psoriatic symptoms and overall quality of life (QoL) [2].

1.1 Psoriasis at a glance

Psoriasis is a chronic, inflammatory, non-contagious and relapsing skin condition with a strong genetic predisposition and autoimmune pathogenic traits [8]. While psoriasis can present at any age, it most commonly appears for the first time between the ages of 15 and 25 years, and then again between ages of 57 to 60 years [9], affecting both men and women equally [3, 10]. The worldwide prevalence is about 2–5% on average, but varies according to regions and ethnicities [3, 10]. In general, the higher or lower the latitude, the higher the prevalence; people from Asian and African countries are less prone to psoriasis than people from regions further from the equator such as Northern Europe, North America and Australia [10, 11].

The term 'psoriasis' encompasses several distinct clinical forms of the disease, the most common and well-known of which is psoriasis vulgaris, also known as plaque psoriasis. Given the ubiquity of psoriasis vulgaris relative to other forms of the disease, our focus in this chapter will be on this particular form.

The pathogenesis of psoriasis is multifactorial, with genetics being a primary contributor, especially in those with early onset of the disease. Many of the candidate genes are either involved in antigen presentation, immune cell signalling and activation, or skin barrier function, suggesting an intricate interplay between dendritic cells, T cells and the main skin cell type, known as keratinocytes [12, 13]. Several other factors can either initiate and/or exacerbate psoriasis flare-ups. These include: (a) trauma induced by various physical, chemical and inflammatory skin disruptions (e.g., abrasions, incisions, rubbing); (b) bacterial (e.g., *Staphylococcus aureus*) and viral infections; (c) the use of certain medications or drugs (e.g., lithium, blood pressure reducing medications); (d) poor lifestyle habits such as excessive alcohol consumption and smoking; and (e) stress [10, 13, 14].

Psoriasis manifests in several distinct clinical forms according to appearance and the body part affected but predominantly presents as well-demarcated salmon pink plaques (dry and piled up skin cells) and/or lesions with silvery-white scale, accompanied by skin tightness, itchiness, a burning sensation and, in severe cases, even bleeding [1, 3, 10, 13, 15]. These plaques typically appear in a symmetrical distribution and affect extensor areas such as the elbows, knees, lower back, limbs, the scalp, tips of the fingers and toes, palms and soles, the fingernails and toenails, and occasionally, the genitals [3, 10, 13–15]. Patients suffering from psoriasis are frequently categorised into two main groups: (1) mild or moderate psoriasis (most common category; affecting 3–10% of total body area) and (2) severe psoriasis (rare; affecting more than 10% of total body area). Such categorisation primarily depends on the following three aspects: (1) the clinical severity score (also known as Psoriasis Area Severity Index—PASI) of the plaques, which is an assessment tool based on the degree of plaque redness, thickness, itchiness and scaling; (2) the percentage of affected body surface area (BSA); and (3) patient QoL [13, 14, 16].

As alluded to in the introduction, psoriasis is not only a skin condition, it also involves multiple organ systems (e.g., cardiovascular, hepatic, respiratory and haematological) and people with psoriasis regularly display a broad spectrum of symptoms and significant co-existing conditions such as obesity, cardiovascular disease, non-alcoholic fatty liver disease, cancer, diabetes and metabolic syndrome, with rates being especially elevated in those with more severe psoriasis [1, 13]. For example, diabetic patients with psoriasis appear to be more likely to require pharmacological management and suffer from micro- and macrovascular diabetes complications than diabetic patients without psoriasis [17].

1.2 Skin barrier alterations in psoriasis

The barrier function of the skin resides in the outermost layer of the epidermis, known as the stratum corneum (SC) and is linked to the protein enriched corneocyte (dead keratinocytes lacking vital cellular organelles) layers and the intercellular membrane lipid matrix mostly composed of ceramides, cholesterol and free fatty acids [18–21]. Corneocytes are continually and efficiently replaced to maintain skin hydration, flexibility and structural integrity, and to repair any perturbation and damage [21]. Continuous exposure to environmental insults such as harsh climatic conditions (e.g., extreme temperatures, wind) and chemicals (e.g., harsh detergents and soaps) can significantly impact the skin's structural and functional properties, which in turn can cause acute or chronic damage of the skin barrier resulting in unfavourable changes in skin morphology and physiology over time [19, 20, 22–24].

Skin dryness is a major underlying problem of the dysfunctional psoriatic skin barrier as it reflects an abnormal and defective desquamation (shedding) process, where corneocytes are shed as visible scales, causing the cosmetically unattractive rough texture associated with dry skin and excessive transepidermal water loss (TEWL), ultimately leading to discomfort and itchiness. Such compromised, dry and fragile skin that is unable to efficiently bind and hold water is also susceptible to the penetration of irritants, allergens and microorganisms that can result in irritation, inflammation and infection [3, 10, 13–15, 19, 20, 22–24].

Normally, healthy skin cells mature and are shed from the skin's surface every 28 to 30 days [25]. However, when psoriasis develops, these skin cells mature much faster, usually in 3 to 6 days, and subsequently move to the skin surface. Due to such a rapid turnover of skin cells, it is possible that even live and healthy cells can reach the surface and accumulate with the dead cells. Instead of being shed, the skin cells pile up, causing the development of thick plaques that are characteristic of psoriasis [14]. There are two main schools of thought as to the exact pathological process that leads to the development of such psoriatic plaques, however, neither of these can stand independently from each other. The first considers psoriasis primarily as an unregulated condition of excessive growth and regeneration of skin cells, characterised by abnormal keratinocyte differentiation and hyperproliferation. Such a problem is simply seen as a 'fault' of the epidermis and its keratinocytes [3, 14, 26]. The second considers psoriasis as an immune-mediated skin condition in which the excessive regeneration of skin cells is secondary to factors produced by the immune system, suggesting that the inflammatory mechanisms are immune-based and most likely initiated and maintained primarily by T cells found within the deeper layer of the skin, the dermis [14, 27, 28]. Given that keratinocytes, dendritic cells and activated T cells are all crucial to the development and persistence of psoriatic plaques, the pathophysiology of psoriasis cannot be explained by the role of a single cell type exclusively – it is likely a dynamic and complex interplay between those cell types. Furthermore, the contribution of each cell type is equally essential in different phases (e.g., initiation, formation, maintenance) of psoriatic alterations. Therefore, the exact sequence of events that lead to the development of psoriatic plaques remains unknown [28].

1.3 Management of psoriasis

Choosing the best management strategy for psoriasis can often be problematic and frustrating for both patients and healthcare professionals, and usually there are several factors to consider: the type, severity and localisation of the condition; the patient's age and medical history; the impact the disease has on QoL; and the patient's expected goals [1]. Before embarking on a management strategy, it is absolutely crucial to establish expectations and goals. The 'ideal' goal would be complete clearance of psoriatic plaques but this is currently not achievable in most patients. Thus, it is necessary to set a minimal target to allow modification of the management strategy if the target is not achieved within a set time [29]. In very basic terms, management for 'generalised' psoriasis follows a 1-2-3 step-ladder approach (**Figure 1**), starting with topical therapies (e.g., topical moisturisers) (Section 1.4) followed by phototherapy and then systemic medications that can include a range of oral drugs and small biologicals [1, 10, 30].

Topical therapy as monotherapy is useful in psoriasis patients with a mild to moderate condition. Topical moisturisers are also used as an adjuvant strategy for moderate to severe psoriasis that is concurrently treated with either phototherapy or systemic medications [10].

Phototherapy represents a second-line defence strategy in the management of psoriasis (**Figure 1**). It involves exposure of the psoriatic skin to ultraviolet (UV) radiation, which can decrease the appearance of plaques on the skin [10, 31]. Many types of phototherapy have been developed and used for the treatment of psoriasis over the last few decades. Broadband ultraviolet B light (BB-UVB, 290–320 nm) was the first such therapy developed, but was later replaced by narrowband ultraviolet B light (NB-UVB, 311 nm) as the latter is more effective than the former. The excimer laser/lamp of 308 nm was next invented and used as a monochromatic (single wavelength) UVB source for psoriasis treatment. The advantage of using excimer is its targeting ability that can spare unaffected skin while providing high doses targeted directly at psoriatic skin [32]. In short, phototherapy acts by causing cutaneous immuno-suppression, slowing down excessive growth of skin cells and altering cytokine expression [10, 31]. The drawbacks to phototherapy include the extensive time investment that is required; usually, three to five therapy sessions per week are needed, with the total therapy period ranging from approximately 2–3 months. Additionally, the response to phototherapy can vary from individual to individual, and there can be health implications to consider, such as the risk of skin cancer [10].

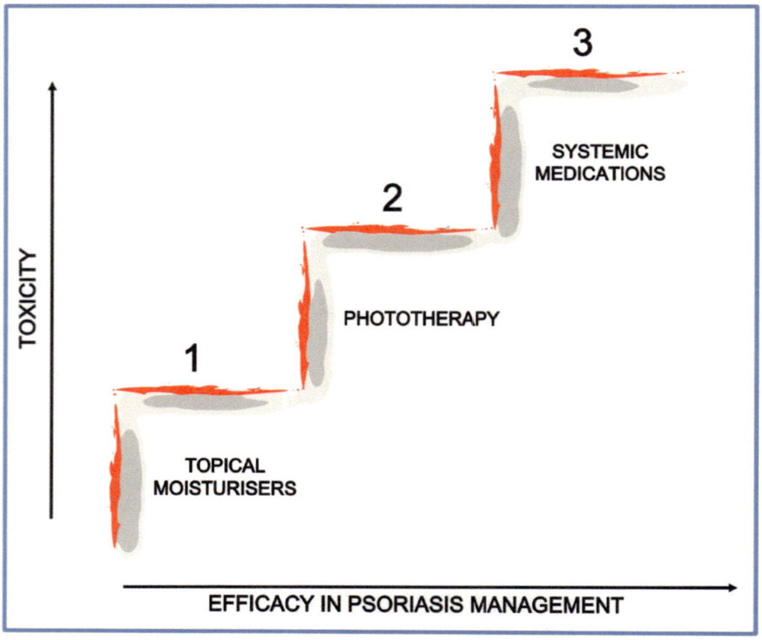

Figure 1.
Schematic of psoriasis 1-2-3 step-ladder management approach [1, 10, 30].

The decision to progress to systemic therapy (**Figure 1**) should be based not only on objective disease severity (where PASI ≥10% or QoL index ≥10% or BSA ≥10%; indicating more than 10% of involvement of the skin) [33], but also on social and psychological factors. The patient should understand the risks (e.g., higher risk and more adverse effects) (**Figure 2**) associated with systemic medications and should be allowed to determine whether the risk of therapy outweighs the benefit [10]. Indications for systemic therapy include widespread plaque psoriasis, erythrodermic (potentially life-threatening inflammation) psoriasis, or the need for repeated hospitalisation for topical therapy. The therapies for extensive and severe forms of psoriasis usually have long-term side effects [34].

The order in which these management strategies are employed should progress in a stepwise fashion from lowest to highest risk (**Figure 2**), hence, the concept of a management ladder (**Figure 1**). The management strategy with the fewest side-effects (e.g., topical moisturisers) should be employed first. If this strategy proves ineffective or if the psoriasis is more severe, strategies with greater toxicity (e.g., phototherapy and systemic medications) may be initiated (**Figure 2**) [10, 34].

1.4 Topical moisturisers are the backbone of psoriasis management

Most topical moisturisers are specifically formulated to promote and maintain healthy skin, but may also serve to manage dry and itchy skin conditions such as psoriasis. Moisturisers are crucial to achieving a reduction in clinical signs of irritation and dryness, scaling and roughness, and a decrease in perceived feelings of tightness and itching [6, 20, 35, 36]. There are no specific rules on what is the best or 'correct' type of topical moisturiser to use. Since topical moisturisers are effectively used either as cosmetics (providing basic skin moisturisation) or therapeutics (e.g., managing psoriasis and preventing its exacerbation), the patients' considerations will be mainly influenced by their personal preferences and lifestyle, and the nature and severity of their skin condition. Individual patient preferences and history may have an impact on the choice of moisturiser or moisturising base to use. A psoriasis patient presenting with severe dryness may benefit most from an occlusive ointment, yet their distaste for this particular base may dissuade them from using the product consistently, which could lead to increased morbidity. Conversely, while a lotion or

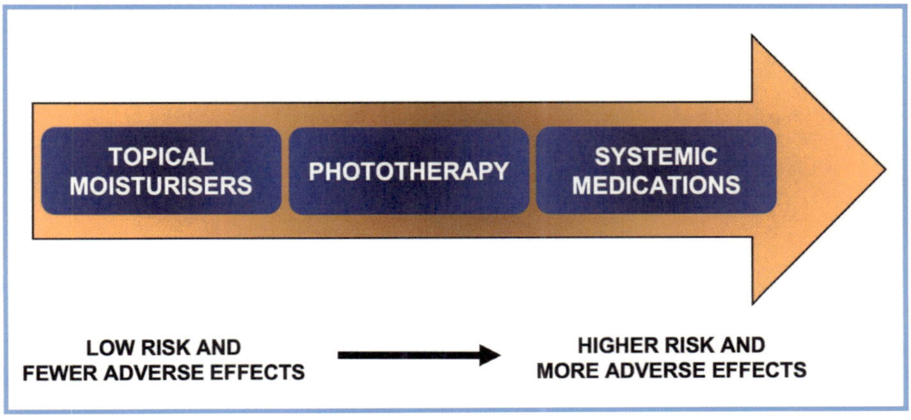

Figure 2.
The order in which management strategies for psoriasis should be implemented [10, 34].

cream may not provide as much hydration as an ointment, the patient's preference for such ingredient base may improve compliance and, therefore, outcome. Patient expectation can also impact the choice or use of moisturiser. Despite wide management options being available, psoriasis is still an incurable disease, so expectation needs to be carefully managed. Complete psoriatic plaque clearance and relief from symptoms is often very difficult, if not impossible, a fact that can lead to patient dissatisfaction, as well as poor adherence and compliance with the current management options [10, 37].

The 'ideal' topical moisturiser (**Figure 3**) is one that the user prefers and will use regularly and liberally, keeping in mind that it should be: (a) cosmetically acceptable and elegant; (b) absorbed rapidly providing immediate skin moisturisation and achieve the intended cosmetic and/or therapeutic effect(s); (c) free from common irritants and allergens such as fragrance, colour and soap to minimise irritation and aggravation of the skin or underlying skin condition; and (d) non-sensitising, non-comedogenic (will not block pores), long-lasting [36, 38] and pH-balanced [39].

The efficacy of topical moisturisers is related to its basic skin moisturisation and 'conditioning' benefits, as well as its therapeutic effects. This is achieved most commonly through a well-designed combination of fundamental and specialty ingredients and actives, formulated and delivered in a range of topical formulations (Section 3) [20, 40, 41].

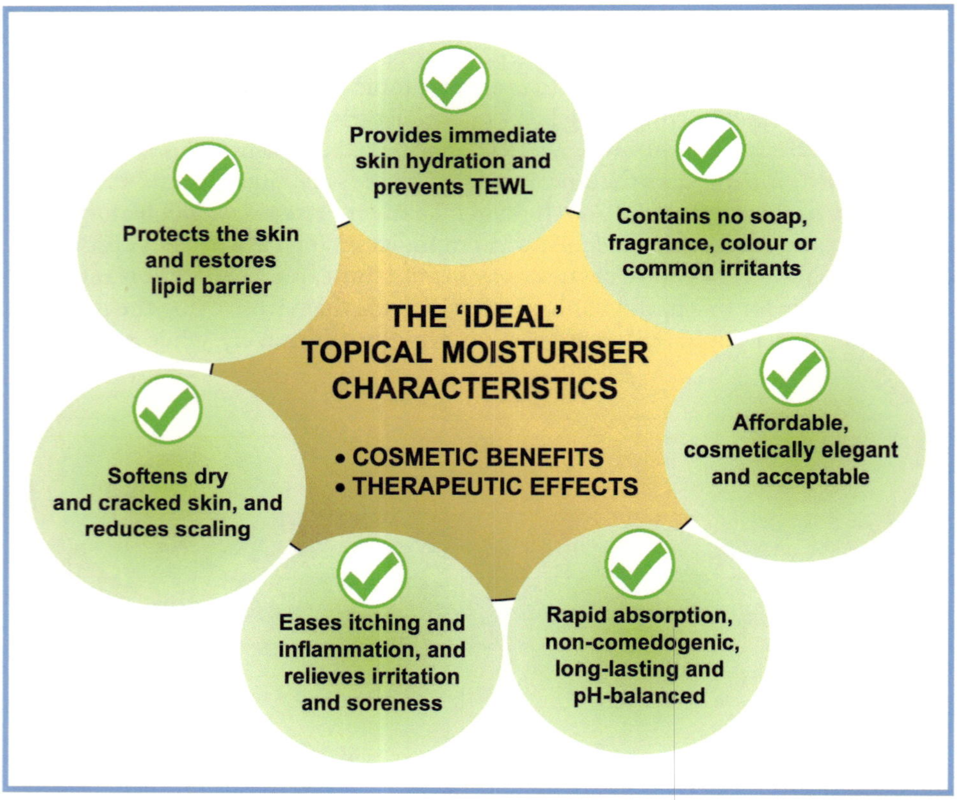

Figure 3.
The 'ideal' topical moisturiser characteristics [36, 38–41].

2. The evolution of moisturisers: from fundamental ingredients to tailored products

The evolution of topical moisturisers is basically equivalent to an odyssey from fundamental ingredients (e.g., emollients, humectants, occludents, excipients) [6, 35, 42] (Section 2.1) to specialty molecules (e.g., ceramides, Panthenol, nicotinamide) [6, 35] (Section 2.2) and functionally distinct actives (e.g., corticosteroids, tar-based ingredients, keratolytics) [43, 44] (Section 2.3). Therefore, understanding the interplay and synergism amongst different ingredients as well as being familiar with their ever expanding biophysical effects is essential to get a cosmetically acceptable and/or therapeutically stable tailored product (Section 3) with the desired impact on both healthy and diseased skin [6, 35].

2.1 Fundamental ingredients

Topical moisturisers usually contain, at a minimum, one or a combination of the key moisturising ingredients, namely emollients (e.g., dimethicone) (Section 2.1.1), humectants (e.g., glycerin) (Section 2.1.2) and occludents (e.g., petrolatum/petroleum jelly) (Section 2.1.3), as well as numerous excipients (e.g., penetration enhancers, preservatives, pH adjusters) to stabilise the formulation (Section 2.1.4). Additional ingredients often include selected specialty ingredients (Section 2.2) and actives (Section 2.3). Ingredient selection, and moisturiser composition and formulation are crucial considerations when choosing an appropriate moisturiser. Specifically for psoriasis, these considerations can determine whether the product will repair and strengthen or further deteriorate the psoriatic skin barrier [6, 35, 45].

2.1.1 Emollients

Emollients are used to improve the appearance and texture of skin by filling in the crevices between corneocytes. This contributes to increased softness, smoothness and suppleness of the skin and improves its overall appearance [42, 46, 47]. The most common types of emollients are silicones such as dimethicone, which is a hypoallergenic and non-comedogenic polymer and is used extensively in topical moisturisers. It exerts a protective effect on the skin by locking in moisture and decreasing TEWL [48]. Dimethicone's low surface energy and highly flexible silicone polymer backbone allows for effective spreading on the skin and a pleasant skin feel. The physical and aesthetic properties of silicones can be controlled by varying the chain length and molecular weight of the polymer. As chain length increases, the viscosity of silicones also increases, and vice-versa. Low viscosity means that the silicone is able to spread quickly and easily while providing a light, silky skin feel, whereas higher viscosities enable silicones to form more persistent hydrophobic (water-repelling) films with good water barrier properties [49].

2.1.2 Humectants

Humectants are hygroscopic (water-attracting) substances that are able to increase the water content of the skin by enhancing water absorption from the underlying skin layers, namely the deeper epidermis and dermis. Humectants penetrate the SC readily and act like biological sponges that promote water retention in the skin [47].

In addition, humectants are also able to hydrate the SC by absorbing water from the external environment. As a consequence, the SC tends to have greater water content in areas in which humectants are localised [42, 46, 47].

Glycerin is the most widely-studied and used humectant. It is also an endogenous component of the human skin. Glycerin is transported from the dermis through the keratinocytes by a transmembrane water/glycerol transport protein, Aquaporin 3 (AQP3) [50–52], and its hygroscopic properties enable it to increase the water holding capacity of an impaired SC. Glycerin functions in a way similar to the skin's own natural moisturising factor (NMF), which is an essential skin process responsible for appropriate SC hydration, barrier homeostasis, desquamation and plasticity. When used topically, glycerin protects the skin from irritant-associated skin conditions and accelerates recovery of irritated skin, while also improving overall skin hydration. Topical glycerin also helps barrier recovery through corneocyte desquamation regulation and is able to restore skin hydration at low usage levels (from as little as 2% v/v up to 10% v/v) [47, 52].

2.1.3 Occludents

Occludents are lipohilic (lipid-loving) substances that form a protective film on the skin and restrict TEWL, trapping water in the skin's uppermost layers and protecting against moisture loss [42, 46, 47, 53]. The most commonly used occludent, petrolatum or petroleum jelly (a long, aliphatic/straight chain of hydrocarbons) [54], can enter the intercellular space of the SC and become part of its lipid structure to provide internal occlusion of the SC, resulting in an increased barrier to water loss. In this regard, petrolatum is often considered to be the most effective moisturising ingredient for dry skin [42, 46, 47, 53].

2.1.4 Excipients

Non-active ingredients, commonly termed excipients, are extensively used in the formulation of topical moisturisers and typically make up the majority (≥90%) of topical product content [41, 55]. By their physicochemical nature, different classes of excipients are used to enhance the functionality of active ingredients in therapeutic products, as well as to aid with formulation challenges. Excipients are often used to: (1) improve solubility to allow incorporation of an active; (2) control the release, penetration and permeation of an active; (3) improve the overall aesthetics of the product to increase patient compliance; (4) improve active and product stability; (5) prevent microbial growth and contamination (e.g., preservatives) and (6) balance the pH of water-based moisturisers, so that they are compatible with the skin's naturally slightly acidic pH [41].

2.1.4.1 Penetration enhancers

Penetration enhancers are chemicals that readily disrupt the structure of the SC and are commonly used to facilitate active (drug) delivery. The cutaneous inflammation experienced by patients with psoriasis promotes hypersensitivity and also suppresses skin barrier function. Therefore, the effective delivery of anti-inflammatory actives such as corticosteroids, aided by appropriate penetration enhancers, can bring about a net improvement in the skin's barrier function [41]. Many penetration enhancers, like propylene glycol, are also solvents, and so can be used alone or in combination with other penetration enhancers to help facilitate both the partitioning into and the passage through the SC. However, care must be taken when selecting and using chemical penetration enhancers since their excessive use can potentially lead to systemic absorption of the active [41, 56]. As such, a careful tradeoff must be made between delivering a therapeutic active dose and protecting the integrity of the skin barrier. Penetration enhancers composed of short chain fatty acids, such as propylene glycol, are thought to integrate into the hydrophilic regions of the packed SC lipids and increase the solubility of this domain for the permeant [41], yet at high concentrations (above 10%) they can irritate the skin [41, 57, 58]. In contrast, penetration enhancers composed of long chain fatty acids like oleic acid insert themselves between the hydrophobic lipid tails to increase the fluidity of the SC lipid bilayers [41].

2.1.4.2 Preservatives

Preservatives are essential components of water-based topical moisturiser formulations and skincare products in general, as they protect products from potentially harmful bacteria. Without preservatives, water-based products would have a very short shelf life and would, for the most part, have to be stored at lower temperatures [59, 60]. Parabens such as methyparaben and propylparaben are arguably the most commonly used preservative ingredients. They have antimicrobial efficacy against a broad spectrum of yeasts, moulds and bacteria, although they are most effective against gram-positive organisms such as *S. aureus* [61]. While parabens exact mechanism of action is not well understood, it is thought to involve the disruption of a pathogen's cell membrane transport processes [62] and the inhibition of DNA/RNA synthesis [63] but it is generally believed that their inhibitory effects on membrane transport and mitochondrial functional processes are key to their antimicrobial actions [64]. The popularity of parabens is based on several advantages when compared to alternative preservatives, including their broad spectrum of antimicrobial activity, stability over a wide temperature and pH range, low degree of systemic toxicity, low frequency of sensitisation, sufficient water solubility, well documented safety record and their lack of odour, taste or colour [59, 60].

2.1.4.3 pH adjusters

In addition to the chemical stability of the ingredients and the formulation itself, pH is a crucial consideration for topical moisturisers. Not only is the absolute pH value important, but the buffer capacity is also crucial to the skin's natural acid mantle. The buffer capacity describes the ability of a formulation to keep the pH value almost constant or as close to the skin's natural pH as possible [65, 66]. This can be achieved by adding pH adjusters to the formulation [66]. The natural pH of the skin surface of most parts of the body is slightly acidic and in the range of pH 4.1–5.8 [66], a feature that can have significant impacts on how the skin reacts to the product. It is a generally accepted fact that the use of alkaline or non pH-balanced products such as soaps, cleansers and creams will lead to skin barrier impairment with a concomitant pH increase in both healthy and diseased skin. The duration of this increase in skin pH depends on skin condition, frequency of application and the composition of the product. Therefore, every skincare product is a potential skin surface pH modifier and the pH of such products must be adjusted to a physiological pH during its development [67]. Some of the most commonly used pH adjusters for topical moisturisers include aminomethyl propanol and citric acid. Aminomethyl propanol is a synthetically produced pH adjuster that is classed as an aliphatic alcohol. It is commonly used in topical formulations due to its safety profile when used in low concentrations [68, 69]. Citric acid is a weak alpha hydroxy acid (AHA) that is naturally occurring in plants and animals. The majority of citric acid comes from citrus fruits, like oranges, lemons, grapefruit and limes. When used and applied in small amounts, it serves as an effective pH adjuster [70].

2.2 Specialty/complimentary ingredients

The newest generation of topical moisturisers for psoriasis also routinely contains specialty or complimentary ingredients in addition to the fundamental moisturiser components detailed in Section 2.1. Common examples of such ingredients include: (1) ceramides that help to replenish the deficient lipids in psoriatic skin [71], (2) the versatile Panthenol (Pro-vitamin B5), which is a skin protectant with moisturising and anti-inflammatory properties [72, 73] and (3) the 'wonder molecule' nicotinamide (also known as niacinamide and Vitamin B3), which is one of the most widely used complimentary ingredients in topical moisturisers [74, 75].

2.2.1 Ceramides

Ceramides, alongside cholesterol and free fatty acids, are the predominant components of the SC and comprise 30–40% of the SC lipid matrix by mass. They are composed of long chain sphingoid bases (e.g., sphingosine) which are linked to long chain free fatty acids. Incorporating the skin's naturally occurring ceramides such as ceramide I (ceramide EOP) and ceramide III (ceramide NP) in topical moisturisers can help to improve both healthy and psoriatic skin by replacing decreased or even depleted ceramide levels [76]. A functional SC plays an indispensable role in ensuring the skin's flexibility and structural integrity. The ordered alignment and organisation of the lipid bilayers within the SC forms a closed system to prevent TEWL in psoriatic plaques and makes the SC more impermeable. Therefore, even a subtle change or disturbance in the amount, physicochemical characteristics and organisation of the SC ceramides can potentially initiate and/or exacerbate psoriasis [71, 77].

2.2.2 Panthenol

Panthenol is a biologically active component of the B vitamin-complex, which is a basic component of the skin, hair and nails. When applied topically, Panthenol is efficiently absorbed into the epidermis and quickly converted into pantothenic acid, which is then converted to Acetyl Coenzyme-A (Acetyl CoA). Acetyl CoA is an essential mediator of many biochemical reactions within skin cells, and is necessary for optimal energy levels, barrier function, moisturisation, elasticity and strength [72, 73]. Furthermore, Panthenol can act as both an emollient and a humectant. As an emollient, it can help seal cracks in the skin, keeping water locked in, which in turn contributes to skin softness and smoothness. As a humectant, it can bind to and hold water effectively, reducing the amount of TEWL through the skin and helping it maintain moisture, softness and elasticity [72, 73, 78].

2.2.3 Nicotinamide

Nicotinamide, which easily penetrates the skin, is fast becoming a ubiquitous topical skincare ingredient in a range of moisturiser formulations. A number of clinical trials [79–81] show that the concentration of topical nicotinamide products can go up to 10%, but desired effects can be achieved with concentrations as low as 2–5% [79]. Nicotinamide provides a long list of skin care benefits with its use, including its ability to: (1) support the skin barrier structure and function by facilitating the formation of ceramides and keratin [74, 75]; (2) improve the skin's tone and texture [82]; and (3) boost the effectiveness of moisturisers in general [75]. For example, when formulated in a combination with glycerin, a nicotinamide-containing moisturiser can very effectively improve the integrity of the SC and thus reduce skin dryness over time [75, 83]. In addition, nicotinamide has also been shown to have anti-inflammatory and antioxidant properties, the latter of which may help to reduce the harmful effects of UV radiation, photoageing and oxidative stress [84]. The appropriate concentration of topical nicotinamide for each individual may depend on their skin type and condition, keeping in mind that in some instances, high levels of nicotinamide can cause an allergic reaction for people susceptible to skin allergies [85].

2.3 Active ingredients

Alongside moisturisers, topical therapeutic products for psoriasis that contain active ingredients can also utilise both the fundamental (Section 2.1) and specialty (Section 2.2) ingredients to compliment the active component of the product or provide additional skin conditioning benefits. Common examples of actives indicated for the management of psoriasis include corticosteroids (e.g., hydrocortisone, clobetasone butyrate, mometasone furoate) (Section 2.3.1), tar-based actives (e.g., coal tar, pine tar) (Section 2.3.2) and keratolytics (e.g., salicylic acid) (Section 2.3.3). While these active ingredients are included to treat specific symptoms or characteristics of psoriasis such as inflammation, itch and plaque build-up, the use of a moisturising base can help to dramatically improve patient outcomes [6, 35]. While non-active moisturisers containing only fundamental ingredients are an important adjuvant therapy of classical psoriasis treatment modalities and used as supportive treatment in relapse-free phases [6, 35, 50], a moisturising base containing a topical corticosteroid will be able to not only manage the inflammation associated with psoriasis but also reduce the dryness and itch, and the accompanying scratch response that can significantly worsen disease morbidity [86].

2.3.1 Corticosteroids

Corticosteroids play a key role in the management of psoriasis. In this context, their mechanism of action involves the reduction of skin redness and the expression of anti-inflammatory mediators, as well as achieving an improvement and/or clearance of psoriatic plaques (**Figure 4**) [87]. These effects are exerted via intracellular corticosteroid receptors, which regulate gene transcription, including several that code for pro-inflammatory mediators. Topical corticosteroids are classified based on their skin vasoconstrictive activity, ranging in strength (potency): (a) super potent/ultrahigh (e.g., clobetasol propionate 0.05%); (b) high (e.g., mometasone furoate 0.1%); (c) moderate (medium) (e.g., betamethasone valerate 0.1%) [43, 86] and (d) low (e.g., hydrocortisone 1.0%) [43]. Choosing a corticosteroid with appropriate

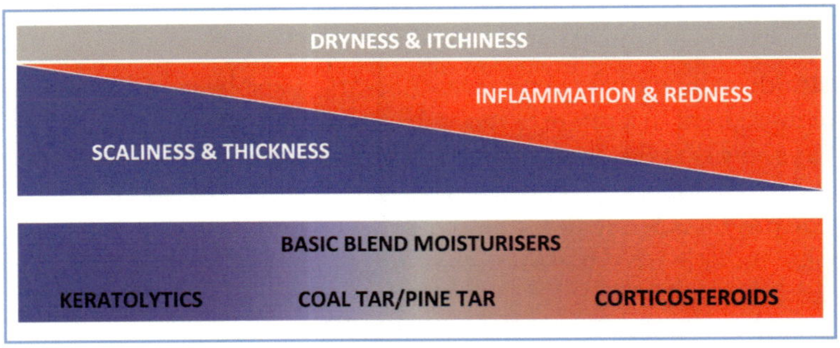

Figure 4.
The choice of management strategy for psoriasis is driven by the skin's dryness and itchiness; inflammation and redness; scaliness and thickness [6, 35, 45, 86, 87, 91, 99].

potency plus the appropriate topical formulation should be based on the disease severity and area affected, and the patient's preference and age [88]. Lower potency corticosteroids such as hydrocortisone should be used on the face, intertriginous areas, and areas that are susceptible to steroid atrophy (e.g., forearms) [88, 89]. In adults, higher potency corticosteroids such as clobetasone butyrate and mometasone furoate are generally recommended as initial therapy [86, 88, 90]. Areas with thick, chronic plaques often require management with ultrahigh-potency corticosteroids. In numerous randomised clinical trials [4, 91–94], different potency topical corticosteroids were effective and safe at 2 to 4 weeks in the management of mild to severe plaque psoriasis. Evidence on the efficacy of topical corticosteroids for the management of psoriasis varies greatly due to the differences in study designs, patient populations, corticosteroid class and concentration, adverse effects and outcomes [86].

2.3.2 Tar-based actives

Tars represent one of the first therapies developed in the history of psoriasis [87]. In fact, pine tar has probably been produced in Scandinavia since the Iron Age and its use in medicine was first described by Hippocrates more than 2000 years ago in ancient Greece to treat a range of skin conditions because of its soothing and antiseptic properties [95]. Pine tar should not be confused with coal tar, which has been produced from coal for approximately a 100 years. Today, it is available in various formulations, from gels, to lotions and soap-free bars [96]. As an effective anti-inflammatory, antibacterial and antifungal substance, topical pine tar has been used in topical formulations for a long time to relieve itchiness and inflammation associated with a range of dry, itchy, flaky or inflamed skin conditions (**Figure 4**), particularly eczema and psoriasis, with minimal safety risk [96]. Furthermore, both coal tar and wood tars such as birch and beech are also available as topical anti-psoriatic ingredients in different topical formulations [87, 97]. Due to its inherent chemical composition and complexity [98], the mechanism of action of coal tar is not well understood, but it likely suppresses DNA synthesis and reduces keratinocyte proliferation. Coal tar is often used as either a monotherapy or in combination with other management strategies [87, 97]. Pine tar is thought to exert its effect by reducing DNA synthesis and mitotic (cell division) activity, which promotes a return to normal keratin development [96]. Tar-based formulations are indicated for the management of chronic, stable forms of plaque-type psoriasis and scalp psoriasis, whereas their use might be limited in sensitive areas such as around the genitals due to their irritation potential [87].

2.3.3 Keratolytics

Keratolytics (**Figure 4**) such as salicylic acid are readily used as active ingredients in many topical formulations, but may have particular utility when it comes to psoriasis as the disease is characterised by a build-up of keratinocytes on the skin. Keratolytics promote the physiologic skin shedding process and also decrease cell-to-cell cohesion in the SC, in effect loosening the glue that keeps keratinocytes together [87, 99]. Salicylic acid has been shown to aid in the removal of excessive keratin in psoriatic plaques and to produce desquamation of the SC while being safe to use and not effecting qualitative or quantitative changes in the structure of the viable epidermis [100]. It is often used as either monotherapy or as part of combination therapy to reduce the size and scale of psoriatic plaques [15, 100]. Keratolytics have proven to be particularly effective in reducing psoriatic plaque thickness if prescribed several days prior starting a first-line treatment (i.e., corticosteroids) for localised psoriasis or in specific areas such as the scalp [87, 99].

3. The necessity of topical moisturiser formulation modality: lotion, gel, cream and ointment

While the specific ingredients used in topical moisturisers or active therapeutics containing moisturising ingredients are important to effectively manage psoriasis, it is equally important to consider the base used to ensure that the product functions as intended. The most common bases include lotions, gels, creams and ointments, and each is distinguished by unique composition and properties that can have significant impact on the cosmetic and/or therapeutic effects they exert on psoriatic skin (**Figure 5**). An important initial factor to consider is the skin's dryness. Very dry skin will likely benefit from an occlusive ointment or cream to trap in moisture, often at the expense of product feel (and as a result, patient compliance) whereas mild to moderately dry skin can often be managed with a lotion or cream, which tend to be more appealing and thus may make for a product that is more readily used. In reality, patients often require more than one topical moisturiser formulation; a less greasy, cosmetically-acceptable product such as a lotion or light cream for use during the day and a heavier or greasier formulation such as an ointment or gel for night-time use [6, 35, 36].

3.1 Combination of basic blend and tailored blend topical moisturisers for the management of psoriasis

The commonly used topical formulation blends, either basic or tailored (**Figure 5**), can provide efficacy through divergent pathways. As these formulation blends contain a unique combination of ingredients (Section 2) they can potentially act through different mechanisms. As a result, there is a scientific rationale for their use in the management of psoriasis, either individually or in combination. This rationale assumes that such formulation blends are selected on the basis of their individual mechanism of action and the biophysical effects they exert on psoriatic skin, which may offer the possibility of synergistic efficacy as well as a reduction in the occurrence of cosmetic problems and side effects (**Figure 6**) [99].

Topical moisturiser formulation blends and topical therapeutics with moisturising bases (**Figure 5**) can be used in a deliberate sequence individually or in combination

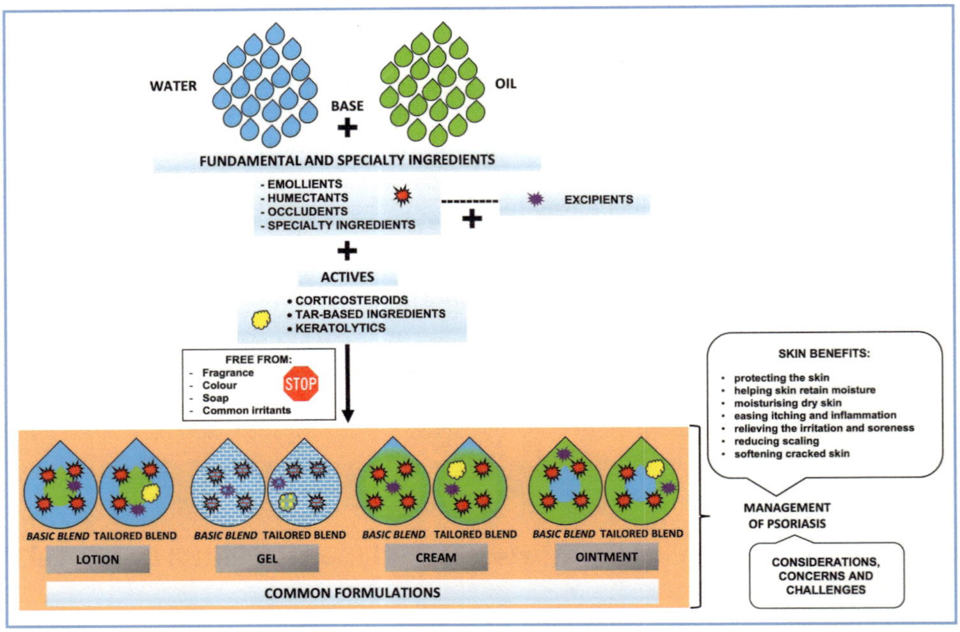

Figure 5.
A range of basic blend and tailored blend topical moisturiser formulations: Lotions, gels, creams and ointments, each distinguished by its unique composition, ingredient combination, and cosmetic and/or therapeutic effects they exert on psoriatic skin, resulting in a range of skin benefits.

	ACTIVE	EFFICACY	RELAPSE RATE	SIDE EFFECTS	COSMETIC PROBLEMS
BASIC BLEND MOISTURISER	-	1	1	0	1
TAILORED BLEND MOISTURISER	Keratolytics	1	1	1	1
	Coal tar/Pine tar	2	1	1	2
	Corticosteroids	3	2	2	0

Figure 6.
Efficacy, relapse rate, side effects and cosmetic problems associated with the use of basic blend moisturisers that contain no actives, tailored blend moisturisers that contain actives such as keratolytics and tar-based actives (coal tar and/or pine tar), and therapeutics with moisturising ingredients and actives such as corticosteroids in the management of psoriasis. Scored on a scale from zero (0) to three (3): 0 denotes little or no change/effect; 3 denotes great and frequent change/effect [102].

(and even with other management options such as phototherapy and systemic medications) with the aim of achieving initial efficacy for the management of psoriasis followed by a safe maintenance regimen. This management strategy maximises the efficacy of each product while helping to minimise relapse rate, cosmetic problems and long term side effects (**Figure 6**) [99, 101, 102].

Now, when we are familiar with a range of basic blend and tailored blend topical moisturiser formulations and their unique composition and ingredient combination (as explained above) (**Figure 5**), an example of a management strategy for psoriasis would be as follows: first, the use of a topical therapeutic with a moisturising base containing a topical steroid potent enough for the severity of the disease (e.g., hydrocortisone for mild, mometasone furoate for moderate to severe) or pine-tar active, at the maximum therapeutic dose, with the main aim of promptly controlling psoriasis flare-ups accompanied by redness and inflammation. This first step can then be followed by the use of a topical moisturiser formulation blend in which a well-tolerated ingredient such as a keratolytic is introduced to reduce psoriatic plaque thickness and scaling. Finally, by using a cosmetically beneficial basic topical moisturiser formulation, the patient can remain indefinitely on a maintenance regimen that aims for continuous hydration of the skin as well as improvements in skin suppleness, flexibility and strength, and the minimisation of dryness and itchiness (**Figure 4**).

While moisturisers are important tools in the management of psoriasis, their use comes with some challenges such as patient perspectives [10] as described in Section 1.4, and some general and more specific concerns regarding the development, uses and regulations of novel anti-psoriatic topical formulations [99]. These include the following amongst many others: (1) heterogeneity in psoriatic plaque thickness, (2) management of psoriasis in different groups of patients (e.g., elderly, pregnant women, children, immuno-compromised patients) requires a few specific care factors and considerations (e.g., prolonged use of topical corticosteroids may lead to thinning of the skin in elderly patients) [10], (3) the safety and efficacy of novel moisturisers when used in combination with existing and established therapies [99] and (4) regulatory requirements and classifications of topical moisturisers, be they cosmetic or therapeutic [103, 104].

4. Conclusions

Psoriasis is a chronic skin condition characterised primarily by dysfunctional skin barrier integrity, dry and itchy skin, and the development of scaly plaques. Being defined as a multifactorial skin condition caused by an interaction between various genetic and environmental factors, psoriasis requires a 1-2-3 step-ladder combination approach of therapeutics to treat the condition and topical moisturisers to alleviate the symptoms.

Therapeutics like topical corticosteroids are not moisturisers themselves, but benefit from having a moisturising base and fundamental and complimentary moisturising ingredients. Therefore, understanding the interplay and synergism amongst different ingredients as well as being familiar with their advantageous biophysical effects and potential adverse effects is essential to get a range of cosmetically acceptable and/or therapeutically stable products with desired impact on both healthy and psoriatic skin.

Topical moisturisers are a key part of psoriasis management and come in various formulations such as lotions, gels, creams and ointments. By using such formulations readily and frequently, the patient can remain on a daily maintenance regimen that aims for continuous hydration of the skin as well as improvements in skin's functionality, structural strength, visual and tactile attributes as well as minimisation of dryness and itchiness.

Conflict of interest

The authors declare no conflict of interest.

Author details

Dalibor Mijaljica, Fabrizio Spada and Ian P. Harrison*
Department of Scientific Affairs, Ego Pharmaceuticals Pty Ltd, Braeside, Victoria, Australia

*Address all correspondence to: ian.harrison@egopharm.com

References

[1] Augustin M, Alvaro-Gracia JM, Bagot M, Hillmann O, van de Kerkhof PC, Kobelt G, et al. A framework for improving the quality of care for people with psoriasis. Journal of the European Academy of Dermatology and Venereology. 2012;**26**(4):1-16. DOI: 10.1111/j.1468-3083.2012.04576.x

[2] Maroto-Morales D, Montero-Vilchez T, Arias-Santiago S. Study of skin barrier function in psoriasis: The impact of emollients. Life (Basel). 2021;**11**(7):651. DOI: 10.3390/life11070651

[3] Rendon A, Schäkel K. Psoriasis pathogenesis and treatment. International Journal of Molecular Sciences. 2019;**20**(6):1475. DOI: 10.3390/ijms20061475

[4] Segaert S, Calzavara-Pinton P, de la Cueva P, Jalili A, Lons Danic D, Pink AE, et al. Long-term topical management of psoriasis: The road ahead. The Journal of Dermatological Treatment. 2020:1-10. DOI: 10.1080/09546634.2020.1729335 [Ahead-of-print]

[5] Lodén M. Barrier recovery and influence of irritant stimuli in skin treated with a moisturizing cream. Contact Dermatitis. 1997;**36**(5):256-260. DOI: 10.1111/j.1600-0536.1997.tb00213.x

[6] Lodén M. Role of topical emollients and moisturizers in the treatment of dry skin barrier disorders. American Journal of Clinical Dermatology. 2003;**4**(11):771-788. DOI: 10.2165/00128071-200304110-00005

[7] Buraczewska I, Berne B, Lindberg M, Törmä H, Lodén M. Changes in skin barrier function following long-term treatment with moisturizers, a randomized controlled trial. The British Journal of Dermatology. 2007;**156**(3):492-498. DOI: 10.1111/j.1365-2133.2006.07685.x

[8] Griffiths CEM, Armstrong AW, Gudjonsson JE, Barker JNWN. Psoriasis. Lancet. 2021;**397**(10281):1301-1315. DOI: 10.1016/S0140-6736(20)32549-6

[9] Griffiths CE, Barker JN. Pathogenesis and clinical features of psoriasis. Lancet. 2007;**370**(9583):263-271. DOI: 10.1016/S0140-6736(07)61128-3

[10] Bakshi H, Nagpal M, Singh M, Dhingra GA, Aggarwal G. Treatment of psoriasis: A comprehensive review of entire therapies. Current Drug Safety. 2020;**15**(2):82-104. DOI: 10.2174/1574886315666200128095958

[11] Gupta R, Debbaneh MG, Liao W. Genetic epidemiology of psoriasis. Current Dermatology Reports. 2014;**3**(1):61-78. DOI: 10.1007/s13671-013-0066-6

[12] Dand N, Mahil SK, Capon F, Smith CH, Simpson MA, Barker JN. Psoriasis and genetics. Acta Dermato-Venereologica. 2020;**100**(3):adv00030. DOI: 10.2340/00015555-3384

[13] Raharja A, Mahil SK, Barker JN. Psoriasis: A brief overview. Clinical Medicine (London, England). 2021;**21**(3):170-173. DOI: 10.7861/clinmed.2021-0257

[14] Kuchekar AB, Pujari RR, Kuchekar SB, Dhole SN, Mule PM. Psoriasis: A comprehensive review. International Journal of Pharmaceutical and Life Sciences. 2011;**2**(6):857-877

[15] Kim WB, Jerome D, Yeung J. Diagnosis and management of psoriasis. Canadian Family Physician. 2017;**63**(4):278-285

[16] Patel RV, Tsui CL. Evaluating psoriasis: A review of the assessments most commonly used in clinical trials. Journal of Psoriasis and Psoriatic Arthritis;**17**(4):259-266. DOI: 10.1177/247553031117a00403

[17] Takeshita J, Grewal S, Langan SM, Mehta NN, Ogdie A, Van Voorhees AS, et al. Psoriasis and comorbid diseases: Epidemiology. Journal of the American Academy of Dermatology. 2017;**76**(3): 377-390. DOI: 10.1016/j.jaad.2016.07.064

[18] Elias PM. Stratum corneum defensive functions: An integrated view. The Journal of Investigative Dermatology. 2005;**125**(2):183-200. DOI: 10.1111/j.0022-202X.2005.23668.x

[19] Lee SH, Jeong SK, Ahn SK. An update of the defensive barrier function of skin. Yonsei Medical Journal. 2006;**47**(3):293-306. DOI: 10.3349/ymj.2006.47.3.293

[20] Roure R, Lanctin M, Nollent V, Bertin C. Methods to assess the protective efficacy of emollients against climatic and chemical aggressors. Dermatology Research and Practice. 2012;**2012**:864734. DOI: 10.1155/2012/864734

[21] Évora AS, Adams MJ, Johnson SA, Zhang Z. Corneocytes: Relationship between structural and biomechanical properties. Skin Pharmacology and Physiology. 2021;**34**(3):146-161. DOI: 10.1159/000513054

[22] Cork MJ, Danby S. Skin barrier breakdown: A renaissance in emollient therapy. The British Journal of Nursing. 2009;**18**(14):872, 874, 876-7. DOI: 10.12968/bjon.2009.18.14.43356.

[23] Agrawal R, Woodfolk JA. Skin barrier defects in atopic dermatitis. Current Allergy and Asthma Reports. 2014;**14**(5):433. DOI: 10.1007/s11882-014-0433-9

[24] Elias PM. Skin barrier function. Current Allergy and Asthma Reports. 2008;**8**(4):299-305. DOI: 10.1007/s11882-008-0048-0

[25] Lawton S. Skin 1: The structure and functions of the skin. Nursing Times. 2019;**115**(12):30-33

[26] Ortonne JP. Aetiology and pathogenesis of psoriasis. The British Journal of Dermatology. 1996;**135**(49): 1-5. DOI: 10.1111/j.1365-2133.1996.tb15660.x

[27] Robert C, Kupper TS. Inflammatory skin diseases, T cells, and immune surveillance. The New England Journal of Medicine. 1999;**341**(24):1817-1828. DOI: 10.1056/NEJM199912093412407

[28] Benhadou F, Mintoff D, Del Marmol V. Psoriasis: Keratinocytes or immune cells—Which is the trigger? Dermatology. 2019;**235**(2):91-100. DOI: 10.1159/000495291

[29] Strober BE, van der Walt JM, Armstrong AW, Bourcier M, Carvalho AVE, Chouela E, et al. Clinical goals and barriers to effective psoriasis care. Dermatol Ther (Heidelb). 2019;**9**(1):5-18. DOI: 10.1007/s13555-018-0279-5

[30] Samarasekera EJ, Smith CH. National Institute of Health and Care Excellence; Royal College of Physicians. Psoriasis: Guidance on assessment and referral. Clinical Medicine (London, England). 2014;**14**(2):178-182. DOI: 10.7861/clinmedicine.14-2-178

[31] Wong T, Hsu L, Liao W. Phototherapy in psoriasis: A review of mechanisms of action. Journal of Cutaneous Medicine and Surgery. 2013;**17**(1):6-12. DOI: 10.2310/7750.2012.11124

[32] Zhang P, Wu MX. A clinical review of phototherapy for psoriasis. Lasers in

Medical Science. 2018;**33**(1):173-180. DOI: 10.1007/s10103-017-2360-1

[33] Gisondi P, Del Giglio M, Girolomoni G. Treatment approaches to moderate to severe psoriasis. International Journal of Molecular Sciences. 2017;**18**(11):2427. DOI: 10.3390/ijms18112427

[34] Lofholm PW. The psoriasis treatment ladder: A clinical overview. Journal of Modern Pharmacy. 2001;**8**(11):12-15. DOI: 10520/AJA16836707_1241

[35] Lodén M. Do moisturizers work? Journal of Cosmetic Dermatology. 2003;**2**(3-4):141-149. DOI: 10.1111/j.1473-2130.2004.00062.x

[36] Kraft JN, Lynde CW. Moisturizers: What they are and a practical approach to product selection. Skin Therapy Letter. 2005;**10**(5):1-8

[37] Feldman SR, Goffe B, Rice G, Mitchell M, Kaur M, Robertson D, et al. The challenge of managing psoriasis: Unmet medical needs and stakeholder perspectives. American Health & Drug Benefits. 2016;**9**(9):504-513

[38] Lynde CW. Moisturizers: What they are and how they work. Skin Therapy Letter. 2001;**6**(13):3-5

[39] Shi VY, Tran K, Lio PA. A comparison of physicochemical properties of a selection of modern moisturizers: Hydrophilic index and pH. Journal of Drugs in Dermatology. 2012;**11**(5):633-636

[40] Mayba JN, Gooderham MJ. A guide to topical vehicle formulations. Journal of Cutaneous Medicine and Surgery. 2018;**22**(2):207-212. DOI: 10.1177/1203475417743234

[41] Danby SG, Draelos ZD, Gold LFS, Cha A, Vlahos B, Aikman L, et al. Vehicles for atopic dermatitis therapies: More than just a placebo. The Journal of Dermatological Treatment. 2020:11-14. DOI: 10.1080/09546634.2020.1789050 [Ahead-of-print]

[42] Nolan K, Marmur E. Moisturizers: Reality and the skin benefits. Dermatologic Therapy. 2012;**25**(3):229-233. DOI: 10.1111/j.1529-8019.2012.01504.x

[43] Uva L, Miguel D, Pinheiro C, Antunes J, Cruz D, Ferreira J, et al. Mechanisms of action of topical corticosteroids in psoriasis. International Journal of Endocrinology. 2012;**2012**:561018. DOI: 10.1155/2012/561018

[44] Reid C, Griffiths CEM. Psoriasis and treatment: Past, present and future aspects. Acta Dermato-Venereologica. 2020;**100**(3):adv00032. DOI: 10.2340/00015555-3386

[45] Purnamawati S, Indrastuti N, Danarti R, Saefudin T. The role of moisturizers in addressing various kinds of dermatitis: A review. Clinical Medicine & Research. 2017;**15**(3-4):75-87. DOI: 10.3121/cmr.2017.1363

[46] Baumann L. Understanding and treating various skin types: The Baumann skin type indicator. Dermatologic Clinics. 2008;**26**(3):359-373. DOI: 10.1016/j.det.2008.03.007

[47] Greive K. Cleansers and moisturisers: The basics. Wound Practice and Research. 2015;**23**(2):76-81

[48] Nair B. Cosmetic ingredients review expert panel. Final report on the safety assessment of stearoxy dimethicone, dimethicone, methicone, amino bispropyl dimethicone, aminopropyl dimethicone, amodimethicone, amodimethicone hydroxystearate,

behenoxy dimethicone, C24-28 alkyl methicone, C30-45 alkyl methicone, C30-45 alkyl dimethicone, cetearyl methicone, cetyl dimethicone, dimethoxysilyl ethylenediaminopropyl dimethicone, hexyl methicone, hydroxypropyldimethicone, stearamidopropyl dimethicone, stearyl dimethicone, stearyl methicone, and vinyldimethicone. International Journal of Toxicology. 2003;**22**(2):11-35. DOI: 10.1080/10915810390204854

[49] Maxon B, Michael SM. Formulating skin care products with silicones: Approaches and strategies. In: Dayan N, editor. Handbook of Formulating Dermal Applications: A Definitive Practical Guide. New Jersey: Wiley and Sons Inc.; 2017. pp. 59-114. DOI: 10.1002/9781119364221.ch4

[50] Fluhr JW, Darlenski R, Surber C. Glycerol and the skin: Holistic approach to its origin and functions. The British Journal of Dermatology. 2008;**159**(1):23-34. DOI: 10.1111/j.1365-2133.2008.08643.x

[51] Caussin J, Rozema E, Gooris GS, Wiechers JW, Pavel S, Bouwstra JA. Hydrophilic and lipophilic moisturisers have similar penetration profiles but different effects on SC water distribution *in vivo*. Experimental Dermatology. 2009;**18**(11):954-961. DOI: 10.1111/j.1600-0625.2009.00881.x

[52] Margolis DJ, Kim B, Apter AJ. Thymic stromal lymphopoietin variation, filaggrin loss of function, and the persistence of atopic dermatitis. AMA Dermatology. 2014;**150**(3):254-259. DOI: 10.1001/jamadermatol.2013.7954

[53] Rawlings AV, Lombard KJ. A review on the extensive skin benefits of mineral oil. International Journal of Cosmetic Science. 2012;**34**(6):511-518. DOI: 10.1111/j.1468-2494.2012.00752.x

[54] Czarnowicki T, Malajian D, Khattri S, Correa da Rosa J, Dutt R, Finney R, et al. Petrolatum: Barrier repair and antimicrobial responses underlying this "inert" moisturizer. The Journal of Allergy and Clinical Immunology. 2016;**137**(4):1091-1102. DOI: 10.1016/j.jaci.2015.08.013

[55] Brown MB, Turner M, Lim ST. Topical product formulation development. In: Benson HAE, Watkinson A, editors. Transdermal and Topical Drug Delivery: Principles and Practice. 1st ed. Hoboken, NJ: Wiley and Sons Inc.; 2012. pp. 255-286. DOI: 10.1002/9781118140505

[56] Parhi R, Suresh P, Mondal S, Kumar PM. Novel penetration enhancers for skin applications: A review. Current Drug Delivery. 2012;**9**(2):219-230. DOI: 10.2174/156720112800234585

[57] Lessmann H, Schnuch A, Geier J, Uter W. Skin-sensitizing and irritant properties of propylene glycol. Contact Dermatitis. 2005;**53**(5):247-259. DOI: 10.1111/j.0105-1873.2005.00693.x

[58] Trommer H, Neubert RHH. Overcoming the stratum corneum: The modulation of skin penetration. A review. Skin Pharmacology and Applied Skin Physiology. 2006;**19**(2):106-121. DOI: 10.1159/000091978

[59] Francisco A, Fonseca AP. Parabens paradoxes in cosmetic formulations; a review. International Journal of Medical Research and Pharmaceutical Sciences. 2016;**3**(8):1-11. DOI: 10.5281/zenodo.61076

[60] Lincho J, Martins RC, Gomes J. Paraben compounds-Part I: An overview of their characteristics, detection, and impacts. Applied Sciences. 2021;**11**(5):2307. DOI: 10.3390/app11052307

[61] Cashman AL, Warshaw EM. Parabens: A review of epidemiology, structure, allergenicity, and hormonal properties. Dermatitis. 2005;**16**(2):57-66. DOI: 10.2310/6620.2005.05008

[62] Freese E, Sheu CW, Galliers E. Function of lipophilic acids as antimicrobial food additives. Nature. 1973;**241**(5388):321-325. DOI: 10.1038/241321a0

[63] Nes IF, Eklund T. The effect of parabens on DNA, RNA and protein synthesis in Escherichia coli and Bacillus subtilis. The Journal of Applied Bacteriology. 1983;**54**(2):237-242. DOI: 10.1111/j.1365-2672.1983.tb02612.x

[64] Tade RS, More MP, Chatap VK, Deshmukh PK, Patil PO. Safety and toxicity assessment of parabens in pharmaceutical and food products. Inventi Rapid: Pharmacy Practice. 2018;**2018**(3):10. DOI: 10.13140/RG.2.2.23621.40161

[65] Wohlrab J, Gebert A. pH and buffer capacity of topical formulations. Current Problems in Dermatology. 2018;**54**:123-131. DOI: 10.1159/000489526

[66] Schulte de Brinke A, Mehlich A, Doberenz C, Janssens-Böcker C. Acidification of the skin and maintenance of the physiological skin pH value by buffered skin care products formulated around pH 4. Journal of Cosmetics, Dermatological Sciences and Applications. 2021;**11**(01):44-57. DOI: 10.4236/jcdsa.2021.111005

[67] Lukić M, Pantelić I, Savić SD. Towards optimal pH of the skin and topical formulations: From the current state of the art to tailored products. Cosmetics. 2021;**8**(3):69. DOI: 10.3390/cosmetics8030069

[68] Burnett CL, Bergfeld WF, Belsito DV, Klaassen CD, Marks JG Jr, Shank RC, et al. Cosmetic ingredient review expert panel, Andersen FA. Final amended report on safety assessment on aminomethyl propanol and aminomethyl propanediol. International Journal of Toxicology. 2009;**28**(6):141S-161S. DOI: 10.1177/1091581809350932

[69] Becker LC, Bergfeld WF, Belsito DV, Hill RA, Klaassen CD, Liebler DC, et al. Safety assessment of tromethamine, aminomethyl propanediol, and aminoethyl propanediol as used in cosmetics. International Journal of Toxicology. 2018;**37**(1):5S-18S. DOI: 10.1177/1091581817738242

[70] Fiume MM, Heldreth BA, Bergfeld WF, Belsito DV, Hill RA, Klaassen CD, et al. Safety assessment of citric acid, inorganic citrate salts, and alkyl citrate esters as used in cosmetics. International Journal of Toxicology. 2014;**33**(2):16S-46S. DOI: 10.1177/1091581814526891

[71] Kahraman E, Kaykın M, Şahin Bektay H, Güngör S. Recent advances on topical application of ceramides to restore barrier function of skin. Cosmetics. 2019;**6**(3):52. DOI: 10.3390/cosmetics6030052

[72] Camargo FB Jr, Gaspar LR, Maia Campos PMBG. Skin moisturizing effects of panthenol-based formulations. Journal of Cosmetic Science. 2011;**62**(4):361-370

[73] Proksch E, de Bony R, Trapp S, Boudon S. Topical use of dexpanthenol: A 70th anniversary article. The Journal of Dermatological Treatment. 2017;**28**(8):766-773. DOI: 10.1080/09546634.2017.1325310

[74] Gehring W. Nicotinic acid/niacinamide and the skin. Journal of Cosmetic Dermatology. 2004;**3**(2):88-93. DOI: 10.1111/j.1473-2130.2004.00115.x

[75] Christman JC, Fix DK, Lucus SC, Watson D, Desmier E, Wilkerson RJ, et al. Two randomized, controlled, comparative studies of the stratum corneum integrity benefits of two cosmetic niacinamide/glycerin body moisturizers vs. conventional body moisturizers. Journal of Drugs in Dermatology. 2012;**11**(1):22-29

[76] Tessema EN, Gebre-Mariam T, Neubert RHH, Wohlrab J. Potential applications of phyto-derived ceramides in improving epidermal barrier function. Skin Pharmacology and Physiology. 2017;**30**(3):115-138. DOI: 10.1159/000464337

[77] Pietrzak A, Michalak-Stoma A, Chodorowska G, Szepietowski JC. Lipid disturbances in psoriasis: An update. Mediators of Inflammation. 2010;**2010**:535612. DOI: 10.1155/2010/535612

[78] Stettler H, Kurka P, Kandzora J, Pavel V, Breuer M, Macura-Biegun A. A new topical panthenol-containing emollient for maintenance treatment of childhood atopic dermatitis: Results from a multicenter prospective study. The Journal of Dermatological Treatment. 2017;**28**(8):774-779. DOI: 10.1080/09546634.2017.1328938

[79] Levin J, Momin SB. How much do we really know about our favorite cosmeceutical ingredients? The Journal of Clinical and Aesthetic Dermatology. 2010;**3**(2):22-41

[80] Forbat E, Al-Niaimi F, Ali FR. Use of nicotinamide in dermatology. Clinical and Experimental Dermatology. 2017;**42**(2):137-144. DOI: 10.1111/ced.13021

[81] Boo YC. Mechanistic basis and clinical evidence for the applications of nicotinamide (niacinamide) to control skin aging and pigmentation. Antioxidants (Basel). 2021;**10**(8):1315. DOI: 10.3390/antiox10081315

[82] Bissett DL, Miyamoto K, Sun P, Li J, Berge CA. Topical niacinamide reduces yellowing, wrinkling, red blotchiness, and hyperpigmented spots in aging facial skin. International Journal of Cosmetic Science. 2004;**26**(5):231-238. DOI: 10.1111/j.1467-2494.2004.00228.x

[83] Lichterfeld A, Hauss A, Surber C, Peters T, Blume-Peytavi U, Kottner J. Evidence-based skin care: A systematic literature review and the development of a basic skin care algorithm. Journal of Wound, Ostomy, and Continence Nursing. 2015;**42**(5):501-524. DOI: 10.1097/WON.0000000000000162

[84] Gensler HL. Prevention of photoimmunosuppression and photocarcinogenesis by topical nicotinamide. Nutrition and Cancer. 1997;**29**(2):157-162. DOI: 10.1080/01635589709514618

[85] Tian YJ, Li D, Ma Q, Gu XY, Guo M, Lun YZ, et al. Excess nicotinamide increases plasma serotonin and histamine levels. Sheng Li Xue Bao. 2013;**65**(1):33-38

[86] Elmets CA, Korman NJ, Prater EF, Wong EB, Rupani RN, Kivelevitch D, et al. Joint AAD-NPF Guidelines of care for the management and treatment of psoriasis with topical therapy and alternative medicine modalities for psoriasis severity measures. Journal of the American Academy of Dermatology. 2021;**84**(2):432-470. DOI: 10.1016/j.jaad.2020.07.087

[87] Chiricozzi A, Pimpinelli N, Ricceri F, Bagnoni G, Bartoli L, Bellini M, et al. Treatment of psoriasis with topical agents: Recommendations from a

Tuscany Consensus. Dermatologic Therapy. 2017;**30**(6):e12549. DOI: 10.1111/dth.12549

[88] Spada F, Barnes TM, Greive KA. Comparative safety and efficacy of topical mometasone furoate with other topical corticosteroids. The Australasian Journal of Dermatology. 2018;**59**(3):e168-e174. DOI: 10.1111/ajd.12762

[89] Greive KA, Barnes TM. Increased bioavailability of hydrocortisone dissolved in a cream base. The Australasian Journal of Dermatology. 2015;**56**(2):e30-e34. DOI: 10.1111/ajd.12128

[90] Ference JD, Last AR. Choosing topical corticosteroids. American Family Physician. 2009;**79**(2):135-140

[91] Castela E, Archier E, Devaux S, Gallini A, Aractingi S, Cribier B, et al. Topical corticosteroids in plaque psoriasis: A systematic review of efficacy and treatment modalities. Journal of the European Academy of Dermatology and Venereology. 2012;**26**(3):36-46. DOI: 10.1111/j.1468-3083.2012.04522.x

[92] Mason AR, Mason J, Cork M, Dooley G, Hancock H. Topical treatments for chronic plaque psoriasis. Cochrane Database of Systematic Reviews. 2013;**3**:CD005028. DOI: 10.1002/14651858.CD005028.pub3

[93] Das A, Panda S. Use of topical corticosteroids in dermatology: An evidence-based approach. Indian Journal of Dermatology. 2017;**62**(3):237-250. DOI: 10.4103/ijd.IJD_169_17

[94] Kleyn EC, Morsman E, Griffin L, Wu JJ, Cm van de Kerkhof P, Gulliver W, et al. Review of international psoriasis guidelines for the treatment of psoriasis: Recommendations for topical corticosteroid treatments. The Journal of Dermatological Treatment. 2019;**30**(4):311-319. DOI: 10.1080/09546634.2019.1620502

[95] Alqahtani EA, Elagib MFA, Al-Yami RH, Abu Hatlah AS, Faragalla AI, Reddy R. Evaluation of antibacterial activity of pine tar on periodontal pathogenic bacteria: An in vitro study. Ethiopian Journal of Health Sciences. 2020;**30**(6):991-998. DOI: 10.4314/ejhs.v30i6.17

[96] Barnes TM, Greive KA. Topical pine tar: History, properties and use as a treatment for common skin conditions. Australian Journal of Dermatology. 2017;**58**(2):80-85. DOI: 10.1111/ajd.12427

[97] Chiricozzi A, Chimenti S. Effective topical agents and emerging perspectives in the treatment of psoriasis. Expert Review of Dermatology. 2012;7(3):283-293. DOI: 10.1586/edm.12.18

[98] Singh RR, Goyal N, Kaur N. Use of coal tar. SSRG International Journal of Civil Engineering. 2015;**2**(3):28-30. DOI: 10.14445/23488352/IJCE-V2I3P108

[99] Mitra A, Atillasoy E. Topical therapies for psoriasis. In: Soung J, Koo B, editors. Psoriasis. Rijeka: Intech Open; 2012. pp. 309-330. DOI: 10.5772/27027

[100] Jacobi A, Mayer A, Augustin M. Keratolytics and emollients and their role in the therapy of psoriasis: A systematic review. Dermatol Ther (Heidelb). 2015;**5**:1-18. DOI: 10.1007/s13555-015-0068-3

[101] Koo J. Systemic sequential therapy of psoriasis: A new paradigm for improved therapeutic results. Journal of the American Academy of Dermatology. 1999;**41**(3 Pt 2):S25-S28. DOI: 10.1016/s0190-9622(99)70363-4

[102] Greaves MW, Weinstein GD. Treatment of psoriasis. The New England Journal of Medicine. 1995;**332**(9):581-589. DOI: 10.1056/NEJM199503023320907

[103] Wohlrab J. Topical preparations and their use in dermatology. Journal der Deutschen Dermatologischen Gesellschaft. 2016;**14**(11):1061-1070. DOI: 10.1111/ddg.13151

[104] Raj RK, Chandrul KK. Regulatory requirements for cosmetics in relation with regulatory authorities in India against US, Europe, Australia and Asean countries. International Journal of Pharma Research and Health Sciences. 2016;**4**(5):1332-1341. DOI: 10.21276/ijprhs.2016.05.01

Chapter 8

Developing Novel Molecular Targeted Therapeutics for Topical Treatment of Psoriasis

Suxing Liu, Di Li and Weikang Tao

Abstract

Psoriasis is a chronic inflammatory skin disorder. The prevalence of psoriasis is estimated at approximately 100 million people worldwide. In mild-to-moderate, as well as moderate-to-severe, psoriasis, 70–80% of patients start with topical agents and continue to use them with other active therapies. This group of patients can benefit from topical treatment with minimal systemic exposure. The expression levels of IL-23 and IL-17 are upregulated in psoriatic skin compared with non-lesional skin, associated with psoriasis pathogenesis. The skin epidermal proliferation and psoriasis are caused by overactive Th17 cells, which are promoted and stabilized by the activated IL-23 receptor, forming part of the positive feedback loop. FDA approved biologics in IL-23/IL-17 axis (ustekinumab, guselkumab, risankizumab, tildrakizumab, ixekizumab, secukinumab and brodalumab) demonstrated superior clinical efficacy in the systemic treatment of moderate-to-severe psoriasis, providing the clinical proof of concept of the IL-23/IL-17 axis as a major immune pathway underlying the pathophysiology of psoriasis. However, due to the large size and poor permeability into skin, biologics are not suitable to deliver via topical route. Current topical treatments of mild-to-moderate psoriasis are corticosteroids and vitamin D analogues, which have limited efficacy with significant side effects so that patients must avoid long-term use. This chapter reviews current molecular targeted therapeutics under development for topical treatment of psoriasis.

Keywords: psoriasis, topical drug, TH17, IL-23, IL-17, small molecule inhibitor

1. Introduction

Psoriasis is a chronic immune cell-mediated inflammatory skin disease characterized by the formation of scaly indurated erythema occurring most commonly on the elbows, knees, scalp, and lower back, but any skin surface can be involved [1]. The highly visible condition greatly affects people's quality of life that can be stigmatizing. People with psoriasis are at an increased risk of developing other chronic and serious health conditions. Comorbidities include psoriatic arthritis, inflammatory bowel disease, hypertension, diabetes, obesity, and depression. The worldwide prevalence of psoriasis is estimated to be 2–4%, rising up to 9.7% in Scandinavian countries [2, 3].

IntechOpen

Psoriasis can be classified into mild, moderate, or severe disease according to the Psoriasis Area and Severity Index (PASI). Treatment choices are often based on the severity of disease: mild disease often managed with topical therapy, and moderate-to-severe disease requiring systemic therapy for control, often with concomitant topical therapy [4–6]. Effects of systemic therapy in synergy with topical agents may help reduce the burden and achieve better quality of life that psoriasis patients deserve. In mild-to-moderate, as well as moderate-to-severe, psoriasis, 70–80% of patients start with topical agents and continue to use them with other active therapies.

Currently, high-potency topical glucocorticoid and vitamin D derivatives are the main treatments for psoriasis [7–9]. Topical glucocorticoids are effective but their use is limited to no more than 2–8 weeks due to their long-term side effects, such as atrophy [10]. This is particularly true in more sensitive areas, such as the face or intertriginous areas. There are numerous reports of low satisfaction for these topical agents [11]. Hence, there remains great unmet medical needs for developing a highly efficacious and safe topical treatment in psoriasis.

2. IL-23/IL-17 axis is a major immune pathway in the development of psoriasis

2.1 Psoriasis is a TH17-driven disease

In psoriatic skin, immune response is overactive. Excess amounts of cytokines were produced, which caused prolonged inflammation and abnormal proliferation of keratinocytes. In recent decades, genetic and immunological studies have made progress in dissecting the mechanisms of psoriasis. Psoriasis was previously thought to be an interferon (IFN)-γ-producing T helper (TH) 1-driven autoimmune inflammatory disease [12, 13]. However, the discovery of TH17 cells shifted the view of psoriasis as an TH17-dependent pathology rather than TH1 cells [12–14].

IFN-γ is increased in serum from psoriasis patients and its mRNA is elevated in skin lesions [15, 16]. It was hypothesized that IFNγ blockade could decrease disease activity due to the appreciation of elevated IFN-γ expression in psoriasis. A neutralized humanized anti-IFN-γ antibody, HuZAF, was developed and tested in two small pilot studies between 2001 and 2003 [17]. In the study that was designed to determine the efficacy of miltidose HuZAF, of all 10 patients treated four times with 10 mg/kg of HuZAF, only 1 patient (10%) achieved a significant clinical response. The expression of CXCL9 was significantly suppressed by HuZAF through week 12. This finding suggests IFN-γ was successfully blocked by HuZAF in these patients since CXCL9 is heavily regulated by IFN-γ. The limited clinical efficacy of IFNγ blockade by HuZAF in patients with psoriasis suggest that infiltration of TH1 cells in psoriatic plaque likely contribute little to the pathogenesis of this disease.

The naive T cells are differentiated into TH1, TH2, TH17, or Treg cells depending on specific cytokines released by antigen-presenting cells and T-cell receptor stimulation and costimulation. The differentiation of TH17 cells are induced by interleukin (IL)-6, transforming growth factor (TGF)-β, and IL-21 [18–20]. Maintenance of TH17 population requires IL-23, a heterodimeric cytokine expressed by macrophages and dendritic cells [21, 22]. The intracellular transcription factors RORγt and STAT3 are also critical in the development of TH17 cells. Binding of IL-23 to IL-23 receptor (IL23R) attracts a heterodimer of kinase JAK2 and TYK2 and induces phosphorylation of STAT3, which enhances RORγ-mediated transcription of IL-17A and IL-17F [23, 24]. TGF-β1 is abundantly expressed in plasma and scales from psoriatic lesions and transgenic mice that overproduce human TGF-β1 in basal keratinocytes exhibit classic signs of psoriasis [25]. Similar observations were made with STAT3, which is overproduced in psoriasis, and its transgenic mice also exhibit psoriasis-like phenotypes [26]. Under the regulation of IL-23, activated TH17 cells in the skin produce high levels of IL-17, which is often referred to as the IL-23/IL-17 axis.

2.2 IL-23 stimulates TH17 cell survival and proliferation

On developing TH17 cells, the expression of IL-23R is induced by intracellular signaling through RORγt and STAT3 and extracellular TGF-β1. The expression of IL-23R then promotes responsiveness to IL-23, which is the key cytokine in the survival and proliferation of TH17 cells [27, 28]. In psoriasis lesions, IL-23 is overproduced by dendritic cells and keratinocytes [29–31].

The importance of IL-23 in psoriasis has been confirmed by genetic studies. Polymorphisms in both subunits of IL-23, IL23A (p19) and IL12B (p40), and IL23R have been reported to be associated with an increased risk of psoriasis in North Americans, Europeans and Asians [32, 33]. A common risk haplotype of IL-23R, proline at amino acid 310 and arginine at amino acid 381, was identified. A single amino acid change from arginine to glutamine at amino acid 381 in IL-23R was found to be protective against psoriasis. Interestingly, this amino acid is located at the JAK2 kinase-binding domain of IL-23R. It is likely the change to glutamine breaks the IL-23R signaling and blocks inflammatory response induced by TH17 cell. In mouse studies, intradermal injection of recombinant IL-23 in normal-appearing skin induces skin inflammation and produces erythematous, thick and scaly skin with histologic features reminiscent of psoriasis [34], and IL-23 deficient mice were resistant to imiquimod-induced psoriasis-like inflammation [35]. Similarly, mice lacking IL-23 are resistant to experimental autoimmune encephalomyelitis (EAE) [21].

IL-23 belongs to the IL-12 family of cytokines and consists of two subunits: p19 and p40. P19 is unique for IL-23 and p40 is shared with IL-12. There are several lines of evidence to demonstrate the central role of IL-23, but not IL-12, in the pathogenesis of psoriasis [14]. The high expression of p19 and p40, but not IL-12 specific p35 expression, was observed in psoriatic lesions as compared to nonlesional skin [36]. Mice lacking the p35 subunit of IL-12 ($Il12a^{-/-}$) or the IL-12-respectific receptor subunit ($Il12rb2^{-/-}$) significantly increased skin inflammation, consistent with the observation in the EAE model of multiple sclerosis that IL-12 knockout mice led to worsening inflammation [21, 37]. In transgenic mice, overexpression of individual subunits of IL-23 leads to inflammation [38, 39]. Ubiquitous transgenic expression of the IL-23 subunit p19 induced a striking phenotype characterized by multiorgan inflammation, runting, infertility and death before 3 month of age [38]. Furthermore, p40 transgenic mice constitutively produce IL-23 (p19/p40), but not IL-12 (p35/p40), in basal keratinocytes by secretion of transgenic p40 with endogenous p19 [39]. p40 transgenic mice cause an inflammatory skin disease, similar to that of intradermal injection of recombinant IL-23 in mice, confirming the provital role of IL-23, but not IL-12, in psoriasis pathogenesis.

2.3 IL-17 is a central proinflammatory effector cytokine in psoriasis

IL-23 is required for autoimmune inflammation mediated by TH17 cells and produces large amounts of IL-17 *in vivo* [40]. IL-23 injection into skin of wild-type mice induces psoriasis-like symptoms, but not in IL-17 knockout mice, and if the wild-type mice are pre-treated with IL-17 antibody, IL-23-induced disease is blocked, suggesting that IL-17 is downstream of IL-23 and critical role in psoriasis pathogenesis [12].

Among six isoforms of IL-17, IL-17A and IL-17F are the most pathogenic in psoriasis [31]. IL-17A is often referred to as IL-17, for which the TH17 cell lineage is named. Besides TH17 cells, a large number of other skin cells also produce IL-17, including γδ T cells, αβ T cells, neutrophils, mast cells, ILC3s and Tc17 cells. Some production is independent of IL-23 [12]. In psoriatic skin, IL-17 expression is higher, and the number of TH17 cells, γδ T cells, Tc17 cells were all greatly increased compared to normal skin [30, 41]. Genes that are up-regulated in keratinocytes treated by IL-17A *in vitro*, are corresponded to the genes up-regulated in psoriasis lesions, and the overlap is bigger than that by TNF-α or IFN-γ [42]. In response to IL-17, keratinocytes produce a variety of antimicrobial peptides (AMPs) and chemokines. They induce flammation and neutrophil recruitment and lead to hyperproliferation of the epidermis and aberrant differentiation of keratinocytes [43].

Even in nonlesional skin from psoriasis patients, expression of IL-17-downstream genes is higher compared to normal skin, and disease severity is significantly correlated with levels of IL-17 and TNF-α in blood. There is also a strong correlation between PASI scores and pathways related to IL-17 [44]. All the evidence suggests that IL-17 is the central effector cytokine in psoriasis.

3. Clinical proof of concept of targeting the IL-23/IL-17 axis for the treatment of plaque psoriasis

Table 1 summarizes biologics approved by the US Food and Drug Administration (FDA) for the systemic treatment of plaque psoriasis [45–48]. These biologics specifically target cytokines and the receptors involved in psoriasis pathogenesis. Treatment with biologics results in a greater efficacy and better safety profile compared to conventional systemic agents that do not target specific components of the immune system, and demonstrates the essential role of the IL-23/IL-17 axis in psoriasis [49, 50].

The first-generation anti-psoriatic biologics targeting cytokines focussed on TNF, an inflammatory cytokine implicated in psoriasis pathogenesis for a long time. High levels of TNF and its receptors (TNFR1 and TNFR2) are expressed in psoriatic lesional skin [51]. Four TNF blockers were approved by the FDA for psoriasis treatment (**Table 1**). TNF inhibition showed good therapeutic efficacy. At week 24, about 50 to 80 percent of patients reached 75% improvement in the psoriasis area and severity index (PASI75), and 10 to 20 percent got PASI100, which means 100% improvement [14]. Infliximab is the most efficacious TNF blocker followed by adalimumab and etanercept [50]. The primary mechanism of action of TNF blockers in improvement of psoriasis treatment is most likely due to its indirect effect on IL-23/IL-17 signaling pathway. The therapeutic effects of TNF blockade are observed to be associated with a strong reduction of IL-17-dependent genes [52]. In addition, TNF induces IL-23 expression in keratinocytes [53]. The exact roles of TNF in the pathogenesis of psoriasis are not yet completely understood.

Nevertheless, TNF is a versatile cytokine that not only involves inflammatory immune responses, but also contributes to cell death, cell cycling and tissue remodeling [54]. TNF blockers are well-known associated risk factors of serious infections,

Drug Class	Target molecule	Therapeutic Agent (Trade name)	Year of FDA approval	Dose and Administration	Other Indications
TNF blocker (biologics)	TNF	Etanercept (Enbrel®)	2004	50 mg twice weekly for 3 months, followed by 50 mg once weekly; S.C. injection	RA; JIA; PsA; AS
		Infliximab (Remicade®)	2006	5 mg/kg at weeks 0, 2, 6 followed by 5 mg/kg every 8 weeks; I.V. infusion	RA; PsA; AS; CD; UC
		Adalimumab (Humira®)	2008	80 mg on day 1 followed by 40 mg every other week; S.C. injection	RA; JIA; PsA; AS; CD; UC; HS; Uveitis
		Certolizumab pegol (Cimzia®)	2018	400 mg every other week; S.C. injection	RA; PsA; AS; CD; non-radio -graphic AS
IL-12/23 antagonist (biologics)	IL-12/23 p40	Ustekinumab (Stelara®)	2009	45 mg or 90 mg at weeks 0, 4, followed by 45 mg or 90 mg every 12 weeks; S.C. injection	PsA; CD; UC
IL-17 antagonist (biologics)	IL-17A	Secukinumab (Cosentyx®)	2015	300 mg at weeks 0, 1, 2, 3, 4, followed by 300 mg every 4 weeks; S.C. injection	PsA; AS; non-radio -graphic AS
		Ixekizumab (Taltz®)	2016	160 mg at week 0; 80 mg every 2 weeks for 3 months, followed by 80 mg every 4 weeks; S.C. injection	PsA; AS; non-radiographic AS
	IL-17RA	Brodalumab (Siliq®-US; Kyntheum®-Europe)	2017	210 mg at weeks 0, 1, 2, followed by 210 mg every 2 weeks; S.C. injection	none
IL-23 antagonist (biologics)	IL-23 p19	Guselkumab (Tremfya®)	2017	100 mg at weeks 0, 4, followed by 100 mg every 8 weeks; S.C. injection	PsA
		Tildrakizumab (Ilumya™)	2018	100 mg at weeks 0, 4, followed by 100 mg every 12 weeks; S.C. injection	none
		Risankizumab (Skyrizi™)	2019	150 mg at weeks 0, 4, followed by 150 mg every 12 weeks; S.C. injection	none

TNF = tumor necrosis factor; IL = interleukin; S.C. = subcutaneous; I.V. = intravenous; RA = rheumatoid arthritis; JIA = juvenile idiopathic arthritis; PsA = psoriatic arthritis; AS = ankylosing spondylitis; CD = crohn's disease; UC = ulcerative colitis; HS = hidradenitis suppurativa.

Table 1.
FDA approved biologics for systemic treatment of moderate-to-severe plaque psoriasis.

such as lower respiratory tract and skin and soft tissue infections like pneumonia and cellulitis [55]. After initial treatment of around 2 weeks, 2% ~ 5% of the patients developed paradoxical psoriasis: new lesions developed or the existing lesions got worse [54]. This side effect also happened when TNF blockers were used to treat other autoimmune diseases, including Crohn's disease and rheumatoid arthritis [53, 56]. It has been reported that IL-17A expression was strong in skin lesions from patients who had paradoxical psoriasis and needed other therapy [57]. This suggests that under some conditions, IL-17 is not down-regulated while blocking TNFα so that skin lesions continue to develop.

After TNF blockers, biologics that directly target the IL-23/IL-17 axis have been developed. The second-generation monoclonal antibody, ustekinumab, is targeting the subunit p40 common to IL-12 and IL-23, blocking signaling of their cognate receptors that induce a nonspecific inhibition of TH1 and TH17 [58, 59]. Ustekinumab has efficacy similar to TNFα inhibitors. It is better than etanercept, but not as good as infliximab. Ustekinumab received FDA approval for the treatment of moderate-to-severe psoriasis in 2009 (**Table 1**).

IL-17 is a central proinflammatory effector cytokine downstream of IL-23 and implicated in the pathogenesis of psoriasis. The third-generation monoclonal antibodies that neutralize IL-17 became available for the treatment of psoriasis (**Table 1**). Secukinumab and ixekizumab are human monoclonal antibodies against IL-17A. Brodalumab is blocking IL-17RA, which is the receptor for IL-17A, IL-17C, IL-17E, IL-17F and IL-17 A/F heterodimers. As IL-17A, IL-17C and IL-17F are all up-regulated in psoriatic skin [31], it is likely that brodalumab would have a better effect. In a study that brodalumab was given to patients who experienced unsuccessful treatment with either secukinumab or ixekizumab, PASI75, PASI90 and PASI100 scores were achieved in 69%, 44% and 28% of patients [60]. In phase III trials, 30–60% of patients treated with IL-17 antagonists reached PASI100 [61–65]. The superior efficacy of IL-17 blockade over neutralizing IL-12/IL23 and blocking TNF has been demonstrated in head-to-head clinical trials of brodalumab versus ustekinumab [62] and ixekizumab versus etanercept [61, 62].

The most common adverse effects of IL-17 antagonists are nasopharyngitis, upper respiratory tract infections, mucocutaneous candidiasis, transient neutropenia and injection site reactions. Mucocutaneous candidiasis observed by IL-17 inhibition or inborn genetic errors of IL-17 gene [66] suggests the innate, protective role of IL-17 against microbial pathogens on the skin. There is a black box warning for brodalumab due to the results from AMAGINE 1 and 2, where four patients committed suicide during the treatment period [64, 65].

IL-23 is known as the master regulator of TH17 cells. A fourth-generation of monoclonal antibodies against p19 subunits of IL-23, guselkumab, tildrakizumab and risankizumab, have been approved for treatment of moderate-to-severe psoriasis (**Table 1**). In contrast to ustekinumab, these biologics target IL-23 by neutralizing the p19 subunit without disrupting the IL-12 signaling pathway. Selectively targeting IL-23p19 provides better efficacy than ustekinumab [50]. IL-23 antagonists can reach a PASI90 in more than 50% of patients, confirming the provital role of IL-23 in the pathogenesis of psoriasis [67–69].

The head-to-head trial of guselkumab versus ustekinumab demonstrates superiority of selectively targeting p19 subunit of IL-23 among patients who had an inadequate response to ustekinumab with similar types of safety profiles [70]. As demonstrated by clinical trial outcomes, double blockade of IL-12 and IL-23 with ustekinumab resulted in lesser disease improvement versus single blockade of IL-23, confirming IL-23, but not IL-12, is a major player in psoriasis.

In addition, IL-23p19 antagonists exhibit significantly higher efficacy compared to all tested TNF blockers while maintaining a favorable safety profile [69, 71]. For example, guselkumab was superior ($p < 0.001$) to adalimumab for PASI90 response at week 48 (76.3% versus 47.9%), respectively. Compared with IL-17 antagonists, guselkumab exhibits a longer duration of therapeutic effect in patients with psoriasis [69]. This is probably because IL-23 is a key driver of TH17 cell differentiation and survival, and an upstream regulator of IL-17A. IL-17 producing cells are dependent on IL-23 for survival. IL-23 stimulates production of not only IL-17, but also other TH17 cytokines (for example, IL-22) by other immune cell types, including γδ T cells.

The most common adverse events with the use of guselkumab and tildrakizumab are nasopharyngitis, upper respiratory tract infections, and headaches [67–69]. In contrast to IL-17 antagonists, the rate of mucocutaneous candidiasis was infrequent and comparable to healthy control subjects.

In conclusion, clinical outcomes of these biologics targeting IL-23p19 and IL17 are a strong argument for the IL-23/IL-17 axis in driving disease pathology. These molecular targeted therapies not only remarkably alleviate symptoms but also provide a deep understanding of the molecular mechanism of psoriatic disease.

4. New targeted therapeutics in development for topical treatment of psoriasis

Targeting a spectrum of inflammatory mediators involved in the pathogenesis of psoriasis will ensure a favorable safety profile and limited side effects. As discussed above, biological treatment, along with evolving systemic therapy, has revolutionized severe psoriasis management. Development of new and effective biologics has made much progress in our understanding of psoriasis immunopathology. Topical therapy implies good compliance for the psoriatic patients, few adverse systemic reactions as compared to systemic medications. However, biologics targeting proinflammatory cytokines are not suitable for topical route delivery due to the large size and poor permeability into skin. Small molecules targeting intracellular signaling pathway have some advantages over biologic agents, particularly the possibility of topical administration, lack of immunogenicity, the simplified synthesis processes, low-cost production, placing these drugs in a very attractive position for future drug discovery and development in topical treatment of psoriasis. New topical targeted therapeutics undergoing efficacy and safety studies are summarized in **Table 2** based on the information available from the website of ClinicalTrials.gov [72].

4.1 RORγ antagonists

RORγt is a master transcription factor of TH17 cells, which activates the transcription of IL-23 receptor gene as well as pro-inflammatory cytokines such as IL-17A, IL-17F, IL-21, and IL-22, and enhances the inflammatory process. Clinical success of biologics in the IL23/IL17 axis suggests that inhibiting RORγ could be an effective alternative therapy for psoriasis.

Vitae Pharmaceuticals (acquired by Allergan, later by Abbvie) developed an orally active RORγt antagonist VTP-43742 for the treatment of autoimmune diseases, including psoriasis through suppression of IL-17A production and down-regulation of the IL-23 receptor [73]. VTP-43742 with high systemic exposure demonstrated a clear signal of efficacy over a short four-week period from a Phase 2a clinical trial

Drug Class	Target molecule	Agent/company	Administration	Highest clinical trial stage	Status
RORγ antagonist (small molecule)	RORγ	GSK2981278 / Glaxosmithkline	Topical	Phase 1/2	Completed (May 2017)
		ESR-114 /Escalier Biosciences B.V.	Topical	Phase 1/2	Completed (June 2019)
JAK inhibitor (small molecule)	pan-JAKs	Tofacitinib (CP-690550)/Pfizer	Topical	Phase 2	Completed (Jul 2009) (Nov 2011) (Sept 2014)
	JAK1/2	Ruxolitinib (Opzelura™)/Incyte	Topical	Phase 2	Completed (Apr 2009) (Apr 2009) (May 2009)
		CT327/Creabilis SA	Topical	Phase 2	Completed (Jan 2011) (Sept 2012)
	TYK2/JAK1	PF-06700841/Pfizer	Topical	Phase 2	Completed (Apr 20, 2021)
DNMT Inhibitor (small molecule)	DNMTs	DUR-928/Durect	Topical	Phase 2	Completed (May 20, 2020)
PDE4 inhibitor (small molecule)	PDE4	AN-2728 (crisaborole)/ Pfizer	Topical	Phase 2	Completed (Mar 2008) (Dec 2008) (June 2010) (June 2011)
		ARQ-151 (roflumilast)/Arcutis Biotherapeutics, Inc.	Topical	Phase 3	Completed (Nov 2020) (Est. Dec 2022)
AhR agonist (small molecule)	AhR	GSK2894512 (Tapinarof, WBI-1001)/ Glaxosmithkline	Topical	Phase 3	Withdrawn (Sept 2018) (The decision is a business decision based on the need to prioritize and focus resources within GSK)
		Tapinarof (WBI-1001, GSK2894512, DMVT-505)/Dermavant Sciences	Topical	Phase 3	Completed (May 2020); FDA acceptance of NDA for Tapinarof in plaque psoriasis

DNMT = DNA methyltransferase; PDE4 = phosphodiesterase-4; AhR = aryl hydrocarbon receptor.

Table 2.
New targeted therapeutics under clinical trials for topical treatment of plaque psoriasis.

in psoriatic patients [74]. It provides a proof of concept of RORγ antagonists for the treatment of psoriasis, consistent with the clinical success of biologics in the IL23/IL17 axis.

Nevertheless, two drug candidates terminated their clinical trials due to potential safety liability. Four patients in the 700 mg VTP-43742 dose group showed reversible transaminase elevations, which led the company to terminate the development of VTP-43742. In addition, Takeda Pharmaceutical Company terminated a phase 1 trial of oral RORγ antagonist TAK828 for evaluation of the safety, tolerability, pharmacokinetics, and pharmacodynamics of escalating multiple doses in healthy volunteers in the United states (NCT02817516). The decision was based on critical non-monitorable toxicology findings in both monkeys and rats, combined with the potential for teratogenicity in humans [75].

RORγ has two isoforms, RORγ1 and RORγ2 (most commonly referred to as RORγt) [76]. RORγt is a differentially spliced isoform of RORγ1, 19 amino acids shorter at N-terminus. The biochemical assay for evaluation of the compounds using LBD of the receptor will result in pan-RORγ antagonists. RORγt is exclusively expressed in a few distinct cell types of the immune system, including Th17, Tc17, γδ T cells and regulatory T cells [43, 77–80] whereas, RORγ1 exhibits oscillatory expression in liver, brown adipose tissue, and kidney [76, 81]. Systemic exposure of the Pan-RORγ antagonists may have off-target effects against the not-intended target, RORγ1, during the treatment of the diseases. In addition, a mouse genetics study indicated that 50% of embryonic RORγ deficient mice developed T-cell lymphoma [82]. Lymphoma was also observed in adult RORγ knockout mice with immune systems intact [83]. The phenotypes of RORγ knockout mice cause concerns of the consequences of systemic treatment of RORγ antagonists in the patients with psoriasis.

Developing RORγ antagonists with the skin-restricted exposure may alleviate the safety risk of systemic exposure while still maintaining similar efficacy as biologics in the IL-23/IL17 pathway, and may provide a new option as topical targeted therapeutics for psoriasis patients. Phase 1 trial of topical RORγ antagonist GSK2981278 for the treatment of psoriasis was not advanced further (**Table 2**) [84]. 0.03%, 0.1%, 0.8% and 4% GSK2981278 ointments were used in the tria, respectively. Across all doses, infiltrate thickness was not altered. Biomarker results did not support that the target was engaged. Although GSK2981278 was shown *in vitro* as a highly potent and selective antagonist of RORγ, the limited *in vivo* efficacy in reduction of epithermal thickness (23% reduction vs. placebo with imiquimod (IMQ) control at 1% GSK2981278 ointment) was observed in IMQ-induced mouse psoriasis-like inflammation model [85]. The skin exposure of GSK2981278 was not disclosed while its systemic exposure in mouse serum was relatively low [85]. It is speculated that insufficient drug exposure at the target site might be one of the reasons for its lacking efficacy in phase 1 trial [84].

More effort was then focused on developing RORγ antagonists in restricted exposure and prolonged action at the skin while being rapidly eliminated from the systemic circulation for topical therapy in psoriasis. ESR114 topical gel is a selective, potent inhibitor of RORγ designed to have its pharmacological activity targeted to the skin with minimal systemic absorption [86]. In 2019, Escalier Biosciences completed a phase I/II trial evaluating ESR-114 topical gel in patients with mild-to-moderate psoriasis in USA and Canada (NCT03630939, **Table 2**). Nevertheless, no trial results were disclosed yet. In addition, it was reported that a novel series of benzimidazole with RORγ antagonistic activity, SHR168442, was developed with desirable skin-restricted PK properties for a topical drug [87]. SHR168442 suppressed the IL-17 gene transcription, and reduced IL-17 cytokine secretion, and, more importantly, achieved skin-restricted exposure suitable for topical delivery. In the IMQ-induced and IL-23-induced psoriasis-like skin inflammation mouse models, SHR168442 ointment exhibited excellent efficacy, which correlated with the reduction of Th17 pathway cytokines, IL-17A, IL-6 and TNFα. This novel RORγ antagonist may represent a new option as topical targeted therapeutics for mild to moderate psoriasis patients. Results from further clinical evaluation of this specific mechanism for the treatment of mild to moderate psoriasis are highly anticipated.

4.2 JAK inhibitors

The Janus kinase–signal transducer and activator of transcription (JAK–STAT) pathway plays a crucial role in intracellular signaling of cytokine of many cellular processes, important in both normal and pathological states of immune-mediated inflammatory diseases [88]. There are four different types of JAK proteins: JAK1, JAK2, JAK3 and TYK2. The IL-23 receptor relies on a heterodimer of JAK2 and TYK2 for signal transduction, thus highlighting the role of JAKs in the pathogenesis of psoriasis and the therapeutic potential of JAK inhibitors in psoriasis. TYK2-deficient mice, as compared to wild-type mice, exhibit significantly reduced ear swelling and less epidermal hyperplasia when injected with IL-23 [89, 90]. In the absence of TYK2, the production of IL-17 and IL-22 and skin infiltration of various immune cells were also impaired. Taken together with the clinical success of biologics blocking either IL-23 or IL-17 signaling (**Table 1**), these results suggest the great potential for JAK inhibitors and, especially, for TYK2 inhibitors in the treatment of psoriasis.

JAK inhibitors are already on the market for rheumatoid arthritis, psoriatic arthritis, and ulcerative colitis [24]. JAK inhibitors have been tested as potential treatments for psoriasis. The first generation of JAK inhibitors target multiple members of the JAK family and thus display a broader effect but also present more side effects. Many JAK inhibitors tested for oral treatment of psoriasis have only been examined in phase II trials except tofacitinib (reached phase III). It is doubtful that they will be tested further. In recent years, selective TYK2 inhibitors have been developed, and several phase III trials are in progress. The highly selective TYK2 inhibitor BMS-986165 has shown high efficacy toward psoriasis, confirming the important role of the IL-23/IL-17 axis in pathogenesis of psoriasis [91]. Several JAK inhibitors with different selectivity spectrums are under clinical development for the topical treatment of psoriasis (**Table 2**).

Tofacitinib (pan-JAK inhibitor) has been approved for the treatment of psoriatic arthritis, but not of psoriasis. Oral tofacitinib has been tested in phase III for psoriasis. Although tofacitinib shows a favorable clinical effect on plaque psoriasis symptoms, herpes zoster occurs during tofacitinib treatment, especially in Asian populations including the Japanese [48]. In phase 2b trial, the ointment formulation of tofacitinib was found to have no considerable effect at week 12 in comparison to that of the vehicle [92].

Ruxolitinib is a selective JAK1 and JAK2 inhibitor that inhibits various cytokines involved in the signaling of TH1 and TH17 pathways, including IL-12, IL-23 and IFNγ, which are associated with psoriasis. Its cream formulation has been approved by FDA for the treatment of atopic dermatitis, but not of psoriasis [93]. In phase II studies, ruxolitinib was studied as a topical ointment for mild-to-moderate psoriasis (**Table 2**). In an open phase 2 study conducted with 28 patients, a greater reduction in lesion severity score was observed for topical ruxolitinib as compared with vehicle and with calcipotriene [94]. The systemic absorption of the product was minimal. In a subsequent phase IIb, double-blind, randomed, vehicle-controlled study, 200 patients with mild-to-moderate chronic plaque psoriasis were treated with topical ruxolitinib for 3 months and the results indicated the mean PASI improvement was 40% compared with placebo [95]. Both studies reported the main adverse event was local irritation, which was more frequent in patients treated with placebo. To date, no phase III study of ruxolitinib in psoriasis has begun yet.

PF-06700841 is a potent dual inhibitor of TYK2 and JAK1, which was shown to be safe and well tolerated in the oral treatment at doses up to 200 mg once daily in a phase I clinical trial [96]. No other clinical trials with oral PF-06700841 in psoriasis are now ongoing. A phase IIb study of topical application of PF-06700841 cream involving patients with mild-to-moderate psoriasis (NCT03850483) was recently completed (April 20, 2021). The trial results are not yet available.

4.3 DNMT inhibitors

DUR-928 is an endogenous sulfated oxysterol that acts as an epigenetic regulator [97]. It binds to and inhibits the activity of DNMTs, DNMT-1, 3a and 3b, inhibiting DNA methylation, and thereby modulating the expression of the genes associated with stress response, lipid biosynthesis and cell death. Improvement of cell survival and reduction of lipotoxicity and inflammation by DUR-928 were observed in animal models and from DURECT's clinical trials in alcohol-associated hepatitis (AH) and nonalcoholic steatohepatitis (NASH). The rationale of topical application of DUR-928 in psoriasis is not clear. A phase IIb study of topical application of DUR-928 topical solution in patients with mild-to-moderate psoriasis (NCT03837743) was completed on August 20, 2020 (**Table 2**). The trial results are not yet disclosed.

4.4 PDE4 inhibitors

The oral phosphodiesterase-4 (PDE4) inhibitor apremilast was approved for the treatment of moderate to severe plaque psoriasis [98]. However, apremilast has only modest efficacy with PASI75 rates clearly lower than biologics. Inhibition of PDE4 indirectly down regulates immune modulators, including TNFα, IFNγ, IL-17 and IL-23 [99]. Due to the potential adverse events associated with oral administration, the topical PDE4 inhibitors, crisaborole and roflumilast, are being investigated as an alternative treatment of psoriasis aiming to avoid systemic adverse effects (**Table 2**).

AN-2728 (crisaborole) ointment has been approved for the treatment of atopic dermatitis [100]. AN-2728 is a newer generation of PDE4 inhibitors [101]. Its binding mode to the catalytic site of PDE4 is distinct from traditional PDE4 inhibitors and can reduce pro-inflammatory cytokines TNFα, IL-2, IFNγ, and IL-5. In phase 2 studies to treat mild-to-moderate plaque-type psoriasis, AN-2728 ointment showed modest efficacy (40% of patients achieved a ≥ 2 grade improvement as assessed by the overall target Plaque Severity Score) [102]. Most adverse effects were mild to moderate.

The oral PDE4 inhibitor roflumilast has been approved by FDA for the treatment of chronic obstructive pulmonary disease (COPD) exacerbation since 2011 [103]. The topical roflumilast, in a high-water-content moisturizing cream base vehicle containing the cosmetic solvent ethoxydiglycol, is being investigated for the treatment of plaque psoriasis [104]. Its inhibitor affinity (IC_{50} values) is 25 to 300 folds more potent than either apremilast or crisaborole depending on PDE4 isoform analyzed [105]. In the phase 2b trial, approximately 85% of the enrolled patients had moderate-to-severe psoriasis and a generally similar percentage of patients in the roflumilast 0.3% group (31%) met the criterion for the PASI75 response at week 8 although differences in trial design do not allow to make direct comparisons [104, 105].

Oral apremilast has been associated with gastrointestinal adverse events of diarrhea and nausea, whereas topical roflumilast cream was associated with less than 1% of each of these events in this phase 2b trial. This may be a result of topical administration bypassing the gastrointestinal tract. Longer and larger trials are in progress to determine the durability and safety of roflumilast in psoriasis (**Table 2**).

4.5 AhR agonists

Tapinarof (also known as WBI-1001, GSK2894512, DMVT-505) is a naturally derived small molecule produced by bacterial symbionts of entomopathogenic nematodes [106]. Broad cellular profiling of tapinatof identified aryl hydrocarbon receptor (AhR) as a primary target [107]. Tapinarof activates the AhR pathway through direct binding. It was reported that AhR activation can modify transcriptional regulation of the immune system and, specifically, affect the differentiation of Th17 and Treg cells [108]. Tapinarof has been shown to inhibit IL-17A message expression by approximately 50% and robustly increase IL-22 levels [107]. Furthermore, 1% tapinarof cream can reduce imiquimod (IMQ)-induced skin inflammation and suppress IMQ-induced IL-17A and IL-17F gene expression in AhR-sufficient, but not AhR-deficient mice.

Topical 1.0% tapinarof met its primary endpoint in patients with mild-to-moderate psoriasis from a randomized double-blind placebo-controlled phase II trial [109]. The improvement in PGA at week 12 was 62.8% for patients randomized to tapinarof when compared with 13.0% for patients randomized to placebo ($p < 0.0001$). The adverse events observed in patients treated with tapinarof were all mild to moderate in intensity.

In 2018, GlaxoSmithKline (GSK) withdrew its phase III trial of tapinarof (GSK2894512) and sold mostly global rights of its Phase III-bound psoriasis candidate tapinarof to Dermavant Sciences [110]. On 9/30/2021, Dermavant Sciences disclosed final results from Phase III PSOARING 3 long-term extension study of tapinarof, a 1.0% once a daily, in patients with plaque psoriasis [111]. 58.2% (302/519) of patients with a PGA score ≥ 2 achieved a PGA score of 0 or 1. Moreover, 40.9% (312/763) of all patients achieved complete disease clearance (PGA score of 0). Those results demonstrate tapinarof's continued improvement in efficacy beyond the 12-week pivotal studies. Treatment-emergent adverse events (TEAEs) were mostly mild to moderate, at application sites, and associated with a low discontinuation rate (5.4%). Incidence and severity of folliculitis and contact dermatitis remained stable with long-term use (up to 52 weeks) and were associated with low discontinuation rates (1.2% and 1.4%, respectively). The FDA accepted the New Drug Application submitted in May 2021, and assigned a Prescription Drug User Fee Act target action date in the second quarter of 2022.

5. Conclusion

A rapidly growing body of literature suggests that the IL-23/IL-17 axis is the major pathway that drives the chronic inflammation underlying psoriasis pathophysiology. The recent years have witnessed that superior clinical efficacy of IL-23/IL-17 pathway biologics in the systemic treatment of psoriasis brings to a major paradigm shift for the management of moderate-to-severe psoriasis. Nevertheless, lack of molecular targeted therapies remains for topical treatment of psoriasis.

With the rapid development of small molecule drugs for the topical treatment of psoriasis, molecular targeted therapies in the IL-23/IL17 axis have the potential to ascertain their role as effective and safe therapy. Although tapinarof and roflumilast are promising therapies in topical treatment of psoriasis, there are still considerable challenges in topical treatment. Many other topical therapeutic agents hold promise and warrant further investigation. Limitations of this chapter include a paucity of randomized controlled clinical trials for topical agents in the treatment of psoriasis, especially for most agents with none or only preliminary data available. Some studies report on a limited duration and a limited number of participants challenging generalizability to the clinic population. Much work is still required for the next breakthrough in the discovery of novel effective and safe topical therapy for psoriasis.

Author details

Suxing Liu[1]*, Di Li[1] and Weikang Tao[2]

1 Eternity Bioscience Inc., Cranbury, NJ, USA

2 Shanghai Hengrui Pharmaceutical Co. Ltd., Shanghai, China

*Address all correspondence to: lius@eternitybioscience.com

References

[1] Griffiths CE, Barker JN. Pathogenesis and clinical features of psoriasis. Lancet. 2007;**370**:263-271. DOI: 10.1016/S0140-6736(07)61128-3

[2] Parisi R, Iskandar IYK, Kontopantelis E, Sugustin M, Griffiths CEM, Ashcroft D. On behalf of the global psoriasis atlas. National, regional, and worldwide epidemiology of psoriasis: Systematic analysis and modeling study. BMJ. 2020;**369**:m1590. DOI: 10.1136/bmj.m1590

[3] Danielsen K, Duvetorp A, Iversen L, Ostergaard M, Seifert O, Tveit KS, et al. Prevalence of psoriasis and psoriatic arthritis and patient perceptions of severity in Sweden, Norway and Denmark: Results from the nordic patient survey of psoriasis and psoriatic arthritis. Acta Dermato-Venereologica. 2019;**99**(1-2):18-25. DOI: 10.2340/00015555-3017

[4] Menter A, Korman NJ, Elmets CA, Feldman SR, Gelfand JM, Gordon KB, et al. Guidelines of care for the management of psoriasis and psoriatic arthritis. Section 3. Guidelines of care for the management and treatment of psoriasis with topical therapies. Journal of the American Academy of Dermatology. 2009;**60**(4):643-659. DOI: 10.1016/j.jaad.2008.12.032

[5] van de Kerkhof PC, Reich K, Kavanaugh A, bachelez H, Barker J, Girolomoni G, et al. Physician perspectives in the management of psoriasis and psoriatic arthritis: Results from the population-based multinational assessment of psoriasis and psoriatic arthritis survey. Journal of the European Academy of Dermatology and Venereology. 2015;**29**(10):2002-2010. DOI: 10.1111/jdv.13150

[6] Boehncke WH, Schon MP. Psoriasis. Lancet. 2015;**386**(9997):983-994. DOI: 10.1016/S0140-6736(14)61909-7

[7] Mason AR, Mason J, Cork M, Dooley G, Hancock H. Topical treatments for chronic plaque psoriasis. Cochrane Database of Systematic Reviews. 2013;**28**(3):CD005028. DOI: 10.1002/14651858.CD005028.pub3

[8] Schlager JG, Rosumeck S, Werner RN, Jacobs A, Schmitt J, Schlager C, et al. Topical treatments for scalp psoriasis. Cochrane Database of Systematic Reviews. 2016;**26**(2):CD009687. DOI: 10.1002/14651858.CD009687.pub2

[9] Maul JT, Anzengruber F, Conrad C, Cozzio A, Hausermann P, Jalili A, et al. Topical treatment of psoriasis vulgaris: The Swiss treatment pathway. Dermatology. 2021;**237**(2):166-178

[10] Coondoo A, Phiske M, Verma S, Lahiri K. Side-effects of topical steroids: A long overdue revisit. Indian Dermatology Online Journal. 2014;**5**(4):416-425. DOI: 10.4103/2229-5178.142483

[11] Oda DC, de Korte J, Sprangers MAG, de Rie M, Smets EMA. Satisfaction with treatment among patients with psoriasis: A web-based survey study. The British Journal of Dermatology. 2013;**169**(2):398-405. DOI: 10.1111/bjd.12372

[12] Blauvelt A. T-helper 17 cells in psoriatic plaques and additional genetic links between IL-23 and psoriasis. The Journal of Investigative Dermatology. 2008;**128**:1064-1067. DOI: 10.1038/jid.2008.85

[13] Fitch E, Harper E, Skorcheva I, Kurtz SE, Blauvelt. Pathophysiology of psoriasis: Recent advances on IL-23 and

Th17 cytokines. Current Rheumatology Reports. 2007;**9**:461-467. DOI: 10.1007/s11926-007-0075-1

[14] Hawkes JE, Yan BY, Chan TC, Krueger JG. Discovery of the IL-23/IL-17 Signaling pathway and the treatment of psoriasis. Journal of Immunology. 2018;**201**(6):1605-1613. DOI: 10.4049/jimmunol.1800013

[15] Uyemura K, Yamamura M, Fivenson DF, Modlin RL, Nickoloff BJ. The cytokine network in lesional and lesion-free psoriatic skin is characterized by a T-helper type I cell-mediated response. The Journal of Investigative Dermatology. 1993;**101**:701-705. DOI: 10.1111/1523-1747.ep12371679

[16] Chodorowska G. Plasma concentrations of IFN-gamma and TNF-alpha in psoriatic patients before and after local treatment with dithranol ointment. Journal of the European Academy of Dermatology and Venereology. 1998;**10**:147-151. DOI: 10.1111/j.1468-3083.1998.tb00715.x

[17] Harden JLLM, Johnson-Huang MF, Chamian E, Lee T, Pearce CL, Leonardi A, et al. Humanized anti-IFN-γ (HuZAF) in the treatment of psoriasis. The Journal of Allergy and Clinical Immunology. 2015;**135**:553-556. DOI: 10.1016/j.jaci.2014.05.046

[18] Bettelli E, Carrier Y, Gao W, Korn T, Strom TB, Pukka M, et al. Reciprocal developmental pathways for the generation of pathogenic effector TH17 and regulatory T cells. Nature. 2006;**441**(7090):235-238. DOI: 10.1038/nature04753

[19] Korn T, Bettelli E, Gao W, Awasthi A, Jager A, Strom TB, et al. IL-21 initiates an alternative pathway to induce proinflammatory T(H)17 cells. Nature. 2007;**448**(7152):484-487. DOI: 10.1038/nature05970

[20] Yang L, Anderson DE, Baecher-Allan C, Hastings WD, Bettelli E, Pukka M, et al. IL-21 and TGF-beta are required for differentiation of human T(H)17 cells. Nature. 2008;**454**(7202):350-352. DOI: 10.1038/nature07021

[21] Cua DJ, Sherlock J, Chen Y, Murphy CA, Joyce B, Seymour B, et al. Interleukin-23 rather than interleukin-12 is the critical cytokine for autoimmune inflammation of the brain. Nature. 2003;**421**(6924):744-748. DOI: 10.1038/nature01355

[22] Langrish CL, Chen Y, Blumenschein WM, Mattson J, Basham B, Sedgwick JD, et al. IL-23 drives a pathogenic T cell population that induces autoimmune inflammation. The Journal of Experimental Medicine. 2005;**201**(2):233-240. DOI: 10.1084/jem.20041257

[23] Chen Z, Laurence A, Kanno Y, Pacher-Zavisin M, Zhu B-M, Tato C, et al. Selective regulatory function of Socs3 in the formation of IL-17-secreting T cells. Proceedings of the National Academy of Sciences of the United States of America. 2006;**103**(21):8137-8142. DOI: 10.1073/pnas.0600666103

[24] Kvist-Hansen A, Hansen PR, Skov L. Systemic treatment of psoriasis with JAK inhibitors: A review. Dermatology and Therapy. 2020;**10**(1):29-42. DOI: 10.1007/s13555-019-00347-w

[25] Li AG, Wang D, Feng XH, Wang XJ. Latent TGFbeta1 overexpression in keratinocytes results in a severe psoriasis-like skin disorder. The EMBO Journal. 2004;**23**:1770-1791. DOI: 10.1038/sj.emboj.7600183

[26] Sano S, Chan KS, Carbajal S, Clifford J, Peavey M, Kiguchi K, et al. Stat3 links activated keratinocytes and immunocytes required for development of psoriasis in a novel transgenic mouse model. Nature Medicine. 2005;**11**:43-49. DOI: 10.1038/nm1162

[27] Stockinger B, Veldhoen M. Differentiation and function of Th17 T cells. Current Opinion in Immunology. 2007;**19**(3):281-286. DOI: 10.1016/j.coi.2007.04.005

[28] Oppmann B, Lesley R, Blom B, Timans JC, Xu Y, Hunte B, et al. Novel p19 protein engages IL-12p40 to form a cytokine, IL-23, with biological activities similar as well as distinct from IL-12. Immunity. 2000;**13**(5):715-725. DOI: 10.1016/s1074-7613(00)00070-4

[29] Piskin G, Sylva-Steenland RM, Bos JD, Teunissen MB. In vitro and in situ expression of IL-23 by keratinocytes in healthy skin and psoriasis lesions: Enhanced expression in psoriatic skin. Journal of Immunology. 2006;**176**(3): 1908-1915. DOI: 10.4049/jimmunol.176.3.1908

[30] Res PC, Piskin G, de Boer OJ, van der Loos CM, Teeling P, Bos JD, et al. Overrepresentation of IL-17A and IL-22 producing CD8 T cells in lesional skin suggests their involvement in the pathogenesis of psoriasis. PLoS One. 2010;**5**(11):e14108. DOI: 10.1371/journal.pone.0014108

[31] Johansen C, Usher PA, Kjellerup RB, Lundsgaard D, Iversen L, Kragballe K. Characterization of the interleukin-17 isoforms and receptors in lesional psoriatic skin. The British Journal of Dermatology. 2009;**160**(2):319-324. DOI: 10.1111/j.1365-2133.2008.08902.x

[32] Nair RP, Duffin KC, Helms C, Ding J, Stuart PE, Goldgar D, et al. Genome-wide scan reveals association of psoriasis with IL-23 and NF-kappaB pathways. Nature Genetics. 2009;**41**(2): 199-204. DOI: 10.1038/ng.311

[33] Cargill M, Schrodi SJ, Chang M, Garcia VE, Brandon R, Callus KP, et al. A large-scale genetic association study confirms IL12B and leads to the identification of IL23R as psoriasis-risk genes. American Journal of Human Genetics. 2007;**80**(2):273-290. DOI: 10.1086/511051

[34] Chan JR, Blumenschein W, Murphy E, Diveu C, Wiekowski M, Abbondanzo S, et al. IL-23 stimulates epidermal hyperplasia via TNF and IL-20R2-dependent mechanisms with implications for psoriasis pathogenesis. The Journal of Experimental Medicine. 2006;**203**:2577-2587. DOI: 10.1084/jem.20060244

[35] van der Fits L, Mourits S, Voerman JSA, Kant M, Boon L, Laman JD, et al. Imiquimod-induced psoriasis-like skin inflammation in mice is mediated via the IL-23/IL-17 axis. Journal of Immunology. 2009;**182**(9):5836-5845. DOI: 10.4049/jimmunol.0802999

[36] Lee E, Trepicchio WL, Oestreicher JL, Pittman D, Wang F, Chanian F, et al. Increased expression of interleukin 23 p19 and p40 in lesional skin of patients with psoriasis vulgaris. The Journal of Experimental Medicine. 2004;**199**:125-130. DOI: 10.1084/jem.20030451

[37] Kulig P, Musiol S, Freiberger SN, Schreiner B, Gyulveszi G, Russo G, et al. IL-12 protects from psoriasiform skin inflammation. Nature Communications. 2016;7:13466. DOI: 10.1038/ncomms13466

[38] Wiekowski MT, Leach MW, Evans EW, Sullivan L, Chen S-C,

Vassileva G, et al. Ubiquitous transgenic expression of the IL-23 subunit p19 induces multiorgan inflammation, runting, infertility, and premature death. Journal of Immunology. 2001;**166**:7563-7570. DOI: 10.4049/jimmunol.166.12.7563

[39] Kopp T, Lenz P, Bello-Fernandez C, Kastelein RA, Kupper TS, Sting G. IL-23 production by secretion of endogenous p19 and transgenic p40 in keratin 14/p40 transgenic mice: Evidence for enhanced cutaneous immunity. Journal of Immunology. 2003;**170**:5438-5444. DOI: 10.4049/jimmunol.170.11.5438

[40] McGeachy MJ, Chen Y, Tato CM, Laurence A, Joyce-Shaikh B, Blumenschein WM, et al. The interleukin 23 receptor is essential for the terminal differentiation of interleukin 17-producing effector T helper cells in vivo. Nature Immunology. 2009;**10**(3):314-324. DOI: 10.1038/ni.1698

[41] Cai Y, Shen X, Ding C, Qi C, Li K, Li X, et al. Pivotal role of dermal IL-17-producing γδ T cells in skin inflammation. Immunity. 2011;**35**(4):596-610. DOI: 10.1016/j.immuni.2011.08.001

[42] Muromoto R, Hirao T, Tawa K, Hirashima K, Kon S, Kital Y, et al. IL-17A plays a central role in the expression of psoriasis signature genes through the induction of IκB-ζ in keratinocytes. International Immunology. 2016;**28**(9):443-452. DOI: 10.1093/intimm/dxw011

[43] Ivanov II, McKenzie BS, Zhou L, Tadokoro CE, Lepelley A, Lafaille JJ, et al. The orphan nuclear receptor RORγt directs the differentiation program of proinflammatory IL-17+ T helper cells. Cell. 2006;**126**:1121-1133. DOI: 10.1016/j.cell.2006.07.035

[44] Chiricozzi A, Suárez-Fariñas M, Fuentes-Duculan J, Cueto I, Li K, Tian S, et al. Increased expression of interleukin-17 pathway genes in nonlesional skin of moderate-to-severe psoriasis vulgaris. The British Journal of Dermatology. 2016;**174**(1):136-145. DOI: 10.1111/bjd.14034

[45] Afonina IS, Nuffel EV, Beyaert R. Immune responses and therapeutic options in psoriasis. Cellular and Molecular Life Sciences. 2021;**78**(6):2709-2727. DOI: 10.1007/s00018-020-03726-1

[46] Stewart J. New treatments for plaque psoriasis–latest FDA approvals. 2021. Available from: https://www.drugs.com/medical-answers/new-drugs-treatment-plaque-psoriasis-3511670/ [Accessed: October 6, 2021]

[47] Yang K, Oak ASW, Elewski BE. Use of IL-23 inhibitors for the treatment of plaque psoriasis and psoriatic arthritis: A comprehensive review. The American Journal of Dermatopathology. 2021;**22**:173-192. DOI: 10.1007/s40257-020-00578-0

[48] Honma M, Hayashi K. Psoriasis: Recent progress in molecular-targeted therapies. The Journal of Dermatology. 2021;**48**(6):761-777. DOI: 10.1111/1346-8138.15727

[49] Ronholt K, Iversen L. Old and new biological therapies for psoriasis. International Journal of Molecular Sciences. 2017;**18**(11):2297. DOI: 10.3390/ijms18112297

[50] ten Bergen LL, Petrovic A, Aarebrot AK, Appel S. The TNF/IL-23/IL17 axis—head-to-head trials comparing different biologics in psoriasis treatment. Scandinavian Journal of Immunology. 2020;**92**:e12946. DOI: 10.1111/sji.12946

[51] Ettehadi P, Greaves MW, Wallach D, Aderka D, Camp RDR. Elevated tumor necrosis factor-alpha (TNF-α) biological-activity in psoriatic skin-lesions. Clinical and Experimental Immunology. 1994;**96**:146-151. DOI: 10.1111/j.1365-2249.1994.tb06244.x

[52] Zaba LC, Suarez-Farina M, Fuentes-Duculan J, Nograles KE, Guttman-Yassky E, Cardinale I, et al. Effective treatment of psoriasis with etanercept is linked to suppression of IL-17 signaling, not immediate response TNF genes. The Journal of Allergy and Clinical Immunology. 2009;**124**:1022-1030. DOI: 10.1016/j.jaci.2009.08.046

[53] Li SJ, Perez-Chada LM, Merola JF. TNF inhibitor-induced psoriasis: Proposed algorithm for treatment and management. Journal of Psoriasis and Psoriatic Arthritis. 2019;**4**(2):70-80. DOI: 10.1177/2475530318810851

[54] Banno T, Gazel A, Blumenberg M. Effects of tumor necrosis factor-alpha (TNF alpha) in epidermal keratinocytes revealed using global transcriptional profiling. The Journal of Biological Chemistry. 2004;**279**:32633-32642. DOI: 10.1074/jbc.M4006422000

[55] Dommasch ED, Abuabara K, Shin DB, Nguyen J, Troxel AB, Gelfand JM. The risk of infection and malignancy with tumor necrosis factor antagonists in adults with psoriatic disease: A systematic review and meta-analysis of randomized controlled trials. Journal of the American Academy of Dermatology. 2011;**64**(6):1035-1050

[56] Mazloom SE, Yan D, Hu JZ, Ya J, Husni ME, Warren CB, et al. TNF-α inhibitor-induced psoriasis: A decade of experience at the Cleveland Clinic. Journal of the American Academy of Dermatology. 2020;**83**(6):1590-1598. DOI: 10.1016/j.jaad.2018.12.018

[57] Tillack C, Ehmann LM, Friedrich M, Laubender RP, Papay P, Vogelsang H, et al. Anti-TNF antibody-induced psoriasiform skin lesions in patients with inflammatory bowel disease are characterised by interferon-γ-expressing Th1 cells and IL-17A/IL-22-expressing Th17 cells and respond to anti-IL-12/IL-23 antibody treatment. Gut. 2014;**63**(4):567-577. DOI: 10.1136/gutjnl-2012-302853

[58] Leonardi CL, Kimball AB, Papp KA, Yielding N, Guzzo C, Wang Y, et al. Efficacy and safety of ustekinumab, a human interleukin-12/23 monoclonal antibody, in patients with psoriasis: 76-week results from a randomised, double-blind, placebo-controlled trial (PHOENIX I). Lancet. 2008;**37**(9624):1665-1674. DOI: 10.1016/S0140-6736(08)60725-4

[59] Griffiths CE, Strober BE, van de Kerkhof P, Ho V, Fidelus-Gort R, Yielding N, et al. Comparison of ustekinumab and etanercept for moderate-to-severe psoriasis. The New England Journal of Medicine. 2010;**362**(2):118-128. DOI: 10.1056/NEJMoa0810652

[60] Kimmel G, Chima M, Kim HJ, Bares J, Yao CJ, Singer G, et al. Brodalumab in the treatment of moderate to severe psoriasis in patients when previous anti-interleukin 17A therapies have failed. Journal of the American Academy of Dermatology. 2019;**81**(3):857-859. DOI: 10.1016/j.jaad.2019.05.007

[61] Gordon KB, Blauvelt A, Papp KA, Langley RG, Luger T, et al. UNCOVER-3 study group. Phase 3 trials of ixekizumab in moderate-to-severe plaque psoriasis. The New England Journal of Medicine.

2016;**375**(4):345-356. DOI: 10.1056/NEJMoa1512711

[62] Griffiths CE, Reich K, Lebwohl M, van de Kerkhof P, Paul C, Menter A, et al. UNCOVER-2 and UNCOVER-3 investigators. Comparison of ixekizumab with etanercept or placebo in moderate-to-severe psoriasis (UNCOVER-2 and UNCOVER-3): Results from two phase 3 randomised trials. Lancet. 2015;**386**:541-551. DOI: 10.1016/S0140-6736(15)60125-8

[63] Langley RG, Elewski BE, Lebwohl M, Reich K, Griffiths CE, Papp K, et al. FIXTURE study group. Secukinumab in plaque psoriasis-results of two phase 3 trials. The New England Journal of Medicine. 2014;**371**:326-338. DOI: 10.1056/NEJMoa1314258

[64] Lebwohl M, Strober B, Menter A, Gordon K, Weglowska J, Puig L. Phase 3 studies comparing brodalumab with ustekinumab in psoriasis. The New England Journal of Medicine. 2015;**373**:1318-1328. DOI: 10.1056/NEJMoa1503824

[65] Papp KA, Reich K, Paul C, Blauvelt A, Baran W, Bolduc C, et al. A prospective phase III, randomised, double-blind, placebo-controlled study of brodalumab in patients with moderate-to-severe plaque psoriasis. The British Journal of Dermatology. 2016;**175**(2):273-286. DOI: 10.1111/bjd.14493

[66] Peul A, Cypowyj S, Bustamante J, Wright JF, Liu L, Lim HK, et al. Chronic mucocutaneous candidiasis in humans with inborn errors of interleukin-17 immunity. Science. 2011;**332**:65-68. DOI: 10.1038/cti.2016.71

[67] Reich K, Armstrong AW, Foley P, Song M, Wasfi Y, Randazzo B, et al. Efficacy and safety of guselkumab,an anti-interleukin-23 monoclonal antibody, compared with adalimumab for the treatment of patients with moderate to severe psoriasis with randomized withdrawal and retreatment: Results from the phase III, double-blind, placebo- and active comparator-controlled VOYAGE 2 trial. Journal of the American Academy of Dermatology. 2017;**76**:418-431. DOI: 10.1016/j.jaad.2016.11.042

[68] Reich K, Papp KA, Blauvelt A, Tyring SK, Sinclair R, Thaci D, et al. Tildrakizumab versus placebo or etanercept for chronic plaque psoriasis (reSURFACE 1 and reSURFACE 2): Results from two randomised controlled, phase 3 trials. Lancet. 2017;**390**:276-288. DOI: 10.1016/S0140-6736(17)31279-5

[69] Blauvelt A, Papp KA, Griffiths CEM, Randazzo B, Wasfi Y, Shen YK, et al. Efficacy and safety of guselkumab, an anti-interleukin-23 monoclonal antibody, compared with adalimumab for the continuous treatment of patients with moderate to severe psoriasis: Results from the phase III, double-blinded, placebo- and active comparator-controlled VOYAGE 1 trial. Journal of the American Academy of Dermatology. 2017;**76**(3):405-417. DOI: 10.1016/j.jaad.2016.11.041

[70] Langley RG, Tsai TF, Flavin S, Song M, Randazzo B, Wasfi Y, et al. Efficacy and safety of guselkumab in patients with psoriasis who have an inadequate response to ustekinumab: Results of the randomized, double-blind, phase III NAVIGATE trial. The British Journal of Dermatology. 2018;**178**:114-123. DOI: 10.1111/bjd.15750

[71] Gordon KB, Duffin KC, Bissonnette R, Prinz JC, Wasfi Y, Li S, et al. A phase 2 trial of guselkumab versus adalimumab for plaque psoriasis.

The New England Journal of Medicine. 2015;**373**(2):136-144. DOI: 10.1056/NEJMoa1501646

[72] Information of the clinical trials. Available from: https://clinicaltrials.gov/ [Accessed: October 22, 2021]

[73] McGeehan GM, Bukhtiyarov Y, Zhao Y, Shi M, Noto P, Stadanlick J, et al. VTP-43742 is a potent and selective RORγt blocker that demonstrates oral efficacy in a mouse model of autoimmunity through suppression of IL-17A production (THER7P.945). Journal of Immunology 2015;194 (Supplement 1) 208.5

[74] Gege C. RORγt inhibitors as potential back-ups for the phase II candidate VTP-43742 from vitae pharmaceuticals: Patent evaluation of WO2016061160 and US20160122345. Expert Opinion on Therapeutic Patents. 2017;**27**:1-8. DOI: 10.1080/13543776.2017.1262350

[75] Takeda. Results for FY2016 Data Book by Takeda Pharmaceutical Company Limited. May 10, 2017. Available from: https://www.takeda.com/siteassets/system/investors/report/quarterlyannouncements/fy2016/fy-2016-q4-announcements-released-on-may-10-2017/qr2016_q4_d1_en.pdf. [Accessed: November 10, 2021]

[76] Jetten AM. Retinoid-related orphan receptors (RORs): Critical roles in development, immunity, circadian rhythm, and cellular metabolism. Nuclear Receptor Signaling. 2009;7:e003. DOI: 10.11131/2015/101185

[77] Ortiz MA, Piedrafita FJ, Pfahl M, Maki R. TOR: A new orphan receptor expressed in the thymus that can modulate retinoid and thyroid hormone signals. Molecular Endocrinology. 1995;**9**(12):1679-1691. DOI: 10.1210/mend.9.12.8614404

[78] Yen HR, Harris TJ, Wada S, Grosso JF, Getnet D, Goldberg MV, et al. Tc17 CD8 T cells: Functional plasticity and subset diversity. Journal of Immunology. 2009;**183**(11):7161-7168. DOI: 10.4049/jimmunol.0900368

[79] Sutton CE, Mielke LA, Mills KH. IL-17-producing γδ T cells and innate lymphoid cells. European Journal of Immunology. 2012;**42**:2221-2231. DOI: 10.1002/eji.201242569

[80] Spits H, Cupedo T. Innate lymphoid cells: Emerging insights in development, lineage relationships, and function. Annual Review of Immunology. 2012;**30**:647-675. DOI: 10.1146/annurev-immunol-020711-075053

[81] Ruan Q, Kameswaran V, Zhang Y, Zheng S, Sun J, Wang J, et al. The Th17 immune response is controlled by the Rel-RORγ-RORγ T transcriptional axis. The Journal of Experimental Medicine. 2011;**208**(11):2321-2333. DOI: 10.1084/jem.20110462

[82] Ueda E, Kurebayashi S, Sakaue M, Backlund M, Koller B, Jetten AM. High incidence of T-cell lymphomas in mice deficient in the retinoid-related orphan receptor RORgamma. Cancer Research. 2002;**62**(3):901-909

[83] Liljevald M, Rehnberg M, Soderberg M, Ramnegard M, Borjesson J, Luciani D, et al. Retinoid-related orphan receptor γ (RORγ) adult induced knockout mice develop lymphoblastic lymphoma. Autoimmunity Reviews. 2016;**15**(11):1062-1070. DOI: 10.1016/j.autrev.2016.07.036

[84] Kang EG, Wu S, Gupta A, von Mackensen YL, Sienerzki H, Freudenberg JM, et al. A phase I randomized controlled trial to evaluate safety and clinical effect of topically applied GSK2981278 ointment in a

psoriasis plaque test. The British Journal of Dermatology. 2017;**178**:1427-1429. DOI: 10.1111/bjd.16131

[85] Smith SH, Peredo CE, Takeda Y, Bui T, Neil J, Rickard D, et al. Development of a topical treatment for psoriasis targeting RORγ: From bench to skin. PLoS One. 2016;**11**(2):e0147979. DOI: 10.1371/journal.pone.0147979

[86] Escalier. Escalies doses first patient with ESR-114 and announces clinical advisory board. 2018. Available from: https://www.prnewswire.com/news-releases/escalier-doses-first-patient-with-esr-114-and-announces-clinical-advisory-board-300695696.html [Accessed: October 13, 2021]

[87] Liu S, Liu D, Shen R, Li D, Hu Q, Yan Y, et al. Discovery of a novel RORγ antagonist with skin-restricted exposure for topical treatment of mild to moderate psoriasis. Scientific Reports. 2021;**11**:9132. DOI: 10.1038/s41598-021-88492-1

[88] Stark GR, Darnell JE Jr. The JAK-STAT pathway at twenty. Immunity. 2012;**36**(4):503-514. DOI: 10.1016/j.immuni.2012.03.013

[89] Ishizaki M, Muromoto R, Akimoto T, Sekine Y, Kon S, Diwan M, et al. Tyk2 is a therapeutic target for psoriasis-like inflammation. International Immunology. 2014;**26**:257-267. DOI: 10.1093/intimm/dxt062

[90] Sohn SJ, Barrett K, Van Abbema A, Chang C, Kohli PB, Kanda H, et al. A restricted role for TYK2 catalytic activity in human cytokine responses revealed by novel TYK2-selective inhibitors. Journal of Immunology. 2013;**191**(5):2205-2216. DOI: 10.4049/jimmunol.1202859

[91] Papp K, Gordon K, Thaci D, Morota A, Gooderham M, Foley P, et al. Phase 2 trial of selective tyrosine kinase 2 inhibition in psoriasis. The New England Journal of Medicine. 2018;**379**(14):1313-1321. DOI: 10.1056/NEJMoa1806382

[92] Papp KA, Bissonnette R, Gooderham M, Feldman SR, Iversen L, Soung J, et al. Treatment of plaque psoriasis with an ointment formulation of the Janus kinase inhibitor, tofacitinib: A phase 2b randomized clinical trial. BMC Dermatology. 2016;**16**(1):15. DOI: 10.1186/s12895-016-0051-4

[93] FDA approves Opzelura. 2021. Available from: https://www.drugs.com/newdrugs/fda-approves-opzelura-ruxolitinib-cream-atopic-dermatitis-ad-5666.html [Accessed: October 22, 2021]

[94] Punwani N, Scherle P, Flores R, Shi J, Liang J, Yeleswaram S, et al. Preliminary clinical activity of a topical JAK1/2 inhibitor in the treatment of psoriasis. Journal of the American Academy of Dermatology. 2012;**67**:658-664. DOI: 10.1016/j.jaad.2011.12.018

[95] Ortiz-Ibanez K, Alsina MM, Munoz-Santos C. Tofacitinib and other kinase inhibitors in the treatment of psoriasis. Actas Dermo-Sifiliográficas. 2013;**104**(4):304-310. DOI: 10.1016/j.adengl.2013.03.002

[96] Banfield C, Scaramozza M, Zhang W, Kieras E, Page KM, Fensome A, et al. The safety, tolerability, pharmacokinetics, and pharmacodynamics of a TYK2/JAK1 inhibitor (PF-06700841) in healthy subjects and patients with plaque psoriasis. Journal of Clinical Pharmacology. 2018;**58**(4):434-447. DOI: 10.1002/jcph.1046

[97] Durect. DUR-928. 2021. Available from: https://www.durect.com/pipeline/dur-928/overview/ [Accessed: October 10, 2021]

[98] Vangipuram R, Alikhan A. Apremilast for the management of moderate to severe plaque psoriasis. Expert Review of Clinical Pharmacology. 2017;**10**(4):349-360. DOI: 10.1080/17512433.2017.1293519

[99] Li H, Zuo J, Tang W. Phosphodiesterase-4 inhibitors for the treatment of inflammatory diseases. Frontiers in Pharmacology. 2018;**9**:1048. DOI: 10.3389/fphar.2018.01048

[100] Pfizer. Pfizer receivers FDA approval for EUCRISA™ (crisaborole), a novel non-steroidal topical ointment for mild to moderate atopic dermatitis (Eczema). 2016. Available from: https://www.pfizer.com/news/press-release/press-release-detail/pfizer_receives_fda_approval_for_eucrisa_crisaborole_a_novel_non_steroidal_topical_ointment_for_mild_to_moderate_atopic_dermatitis_eczema. [Accessed: October 12, 2021]

[101] Akama T, Baker SJ, Zhang YK, Hernandez V, Zhou H, Sanders V, et al. Discovery and structure-activity study of a novel benzoxaborole anti-inflammatory agent (AN2728) for the potential topical treatment of psoriasis and atopic dermatitis. Bioorganic & Medicinal Chemistry Letters. 2009;**19**:2129-2132. DOI: 10.1016/j.bmcl.2009.03.007

[102] Moustafa F, Feldman SR. A review of phosphodiesterase-inhibition and the potential role for Phosphodiesterase-4 inhibitors in clinical dermatology. Dermatology Online Journal. 2014;**20**(5):1. DOI: 10.5070/D3205022608

[103] Oba Y, Lone NA. Efficacy and safety of roflumilast in patients with chronic obstructive pulmonary disease: A systematic review and meta-analysis. Therapeutic Advances in Respiratory Disease. 2012;**7**(1):13-24. DOI: 10.1177/1753465812466167

[104] Lebwohl MG, Papp KA, Gold LS, Gooderham MJ, Kircik LH, Draelos ZD. Trial of Roflumilast cream for chronic plaque psoriasis. The New England Journal of Medicine. 2020;**383**:229-239. DOI: 10.1056/NEJMoa2000073

[105] Milakovic M, Gooderham MJ. Phosphodiesterase-4 inhibition in psoriasis. Psoriasis. 2021;**11**:21-29. DOI: 10.2147/PTT.S303634

[106] Richardson WH, Schmidt TM, Nealson KH. Identification of an anthraquinone pigment and a hydroxystilbene antibiotic from Xenorhabdus luminescens. Applied and Environmental Microbiology. 1988;**54**(6):1602-1605. DOI: 10.1128/aem.54.6.1602-1605.1988

[107] Smith SH, Jayawickreme C, Rickard DJ, Nicodeme E, Bui T, Simmons C, et al. Tapinarof is a natural AhR agonist that resolves skin inflammation in mice and humans. The Journal of Investigative Dermatology. 2017;**137**(10):2110-2119. DOI: 10.1016/j.jid.2017.05.004

[108] Veldhoen M, Hirota K, Westendorf AM, Buer J, Dumoutier L, Renauld JC, et al. The aryl hydrocarbon receptor links TH17-cell-mediated autoimmunity to environmental toxins. Nature. 2008;**453**:106-109. DOI: 10.1038/nature06881

[109] Bissonnette R, Bolduc C, Maari C, Nigen S, Webster JM, Tang L, et al. Efficacy and safety of topical WBI-1001 in patients with mild to moderate psoriasis: Results from a randomized double-blind placebo-controlled, phase II trials. Journal of the European Academy of Dermatology and Venereology. 2012;**26**:1516-1521. DOI: 10.1111/j.1468-3083.2011.04332.x

[110] GSK. GSK sells psoriasis/Dermatitis candidate tapinarof to Dermavant.

2018. Available from: https://www.genengnews.com/topics/drug-discovery/gsk-sells-psoriasis-dermatitis-candidate-tapinarof-to-dermavant/ [Accessed: October 12, 2021]

[111] Dermavant. Dermavant showcases new long-term data from Phase 3 +-PSOARING 3 trial of tapinarof in patients with plaque psoriasis at the 30th EADV Virtual Congress. 2021. Available from: https://www.dermavant.com/dermavant-showcases-new-long-term-data-from-phase-3-psoaring-3-trial-at-the-30th-eadv-virtual-congress/ [Accessed: October 12, 2021]